RECENT ADVANCES IN MICROBIOLOGY

WEST NILE VIRUS

OUTBREAKS, CONTROL AND PREVENTION STRATEGIES

RECENT ADVANCES IN MICROBIOLOGY

Additional books in this series can be found on Nova's website under the Series tab.

VIROLOGY RESEARCH PROGRESS

Additional e-books in this series can be found on Nova's website under the e-book tab.

RECENT ADVANCES IN MICROBIOLOGY

WEST NILE VIRUS

OUTBREAKS, CONTROL AND PREVENTION STRATEGIES

MARINKE VAN VERSEVELD
EDITOR

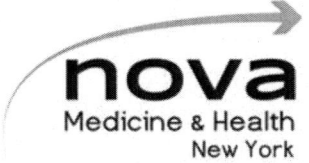

Copyright © 2019 by Nova Science Publishers, Inc.

All rights reserved. No part of this book may be reproduced, stored in a retrieval system or transmitted in any form or by any means: electronic, electrostatic, magnetic, tape, mechanical photocopying, recording or otherwise without the written permission of the Publisher.

We have partnered with Copyright Clearance Center to make it easy for you to obtain permissions to reuse content from this publication. Simply navigate to this publication's page on Nova's website and locate the "Get Permission" button below the title description. This button is linked directly to the title's permission page on copyright.com. Alternatively, you can visit copyright.com and search by title, ISBN, or ISSN.

For further questions about using the service on copyright.com, please contact:
Copyright Clearance Center
Phone: +1-(978) 750-8400   Fax: +1-(978) 750-4470   E-mail: info@copyright.com.

NOTICE TO THE READER

The Publisher has taken reasonable care in the preparation of this book, but makes no expressed or implied warranty of any kind and assumes no responsibility for any errors or omissions. No liability is assumed for incidental or consequential damages in connection with or arising out of information contained in this book. The Publisher shall not be liable for any special, consequential, or exemplary damages resulting, in whole or in part, from the readers' use of, or reliance upon, this material. Any parts of this book based on government reports are so indicated and copyright is claimed for those parts to the extent applicable to compilations of such works.

Independent verification should be sought for any data, advice or recommendations contained in this book. In addition, no responsibility is assumed by the Publisher for any injury and/or damage to persons or property arising from any methods, products, instructions, ideas or otherwise contained in this publication.

This publication is designed to provide accurate and authoritative information with regard to the subject matter covered herein. It is sold with the clear understanding that the Publisher is not engaged in rendering legal or any other professional services. If legal or any other expert assistance is required, the services of a competent person should be sought. FROM A DECLARATION OF PARTICIPANTS JOINTLY ADOPTED BY A COMMITTEE OF THE AMERICAN BAR ASSOCIATION AND A COMMITTEE OF PUBLISHERS.

Additional color graphics may be available in the e-book version of this book.

Library of Congress Cataloging-in-Publication Data

ISBN: 978-1-53616-589-0

Published by Nova Science Publishers, Inc. † New York

CONTENTS

Preface		vii
Chatper 1	Multi-Species, Climate-Driven and Landscape-Based Cellular Difference Equation Model for West Nile Virus: Toward an Agent-Based Model of West Nile Virus Spread *Marcia R. Friesen and Robert D. McLeod*	1
Chapter 2	Recombinant Envelope Domain III Protein of West Nile Virus: Recent Developments and Applications *Nagesh K. Tripathi and Ambuj Shrivastava*	67
Chapter 3	Impacts of West Nile Virus on the Yellow-Billed Magpie and Other Birds in California's Central Valley *Edward R. Pandolfino*	93
Index		109
Related Nova Publications		113

PREFACE

The opening study included in West Nile Virus: Outbreaks, Control and Prevention Strategies aims to design and implement an efficient data-driven agent-based model of West Nile virus spread, considering highly-mobile humans with a high level of heterogeneous properties. The authors propose a cellular difference equation model for adoption in West Nile virus-agent-based models.

Following this, the authors summarize the envelope domain III protein, its production using various host systems, and applications in the development of West Nile virus vaccines and diagnostics.

Lastly, this collection reviews the impacts of West Nile virus on several bird species, and discusses the implications for the long-term survival the Yellow-billed Magpie.

Chapter 1 - The objective of this study is to design and implement an efficient data-driven Agent-Based Model (ABM) of West Nile Virus (WNV) spread, considering highly-mobile humans with a high level of heterogeneous properties. The undeniable value of such an ABM is in simulating and assessing virtually all epidemiological scenarios and prevention strategies. This chapter proposes a Cellular Difference Equation (CDiffE) model for adoption in WNV-ABMs. The proposed CDiffE Model includes multiple species of birds and humans as hosts for the spread of WNV in Southern Manitoba. The migration patterns of different bird species, nocturnal biting activities of *Culex tarsalis* mosquitoes, daily temperature and rainfall, and land cover impact are incorporated into the model. WNV-related parameters for different bird species are estimated according to biological studies on avian viremia. The proposed CDiffE updates on an hourly step in order to act as an environment for a comprehensive agent-based model of WNV spread among peripatetic humans. In general, the model predicts mosquito distribution across the province effectively well. The mosquito population trends within the model over 15 weeks in approximately 30 communities of Manitoba has Pearson and Spearman correlation values of approximately 60% compared with the real-world mosquito trap data. The difference equations are principally much faster than commonly used differential equation models. While the whole system is designed from an agent-based modelling perspective at a cellular level, it exhibits biologically compatible behaviour at the macro-level scale. The geographical output of the current model can be considered a decision support tool for public health policymakers by providing risk maps of mosquito densities. In varying the model parameters, some theoretically verified as well as counter-intuitive findings were observed.

Chapter 2 - West Nile virus (WNV), a mosquito-borne, single-stranded, positive-sense flavivirus, has been linked to acute viral encephalitis and neurological sequelae. Currently neither any antiviral drugs nor any vaccines are licensed for human use. Recent developments on recombinant proteins have paved the way to produce various viral proteins which have potential to be used as diagnostic or vaccine candidates. These recombinant viral proteins are generally produced in microbial and higher expression host systems such as bacteria, insect cells, and transgenic plants. The genome of West Nile virus encodes three structural proteins [capsid (C) protein, pre-membrane (prM) protein and envelope (E) protein) and seven non-structural (NS1, NS2A, NS2B, NS3, NS4A, NS4B, NS5) proteins. The envelope (E) protein has three domains (Domain I, II and III) and it mediates viral binding to cellular receptors and has fusogenic property with the host cell membrane. The domain III (DIII) of E protein contains the neutralizing epitopes that induce strong host antibody responses and provide protective immunity. Due to these reasons, the domain III of E protein can be utilized as recombinant protein vaccine candidate as well as diagnostic intermediate for WNV. In this chapter, the authors summarize about the the envelope domain III (EDIII) protein, its production using various host systems and applications in the development of WNV vaccines and diagnostics.

Chapter 3 - Following the first major West Nile virus (WNV) outbreaks in the Central Valley of California (CV) in 2004-05, local populations of the Yellow-billed Magpie (*Pica nuttalli*) and several other bird species declined significantly. Magpie numbers declined to approximately one-half of their pre-WNV levels. Populations of several other birds, including the Loggerhead Shrike (*Lanius ludovicianus*), California Scrub-Jay (*Aphelocoma californica*), American Crow (*Corvus brachyrhynchos*), Oak Titmouse (*Baeolophus inornatus*), and House Finch (*Haemorhous mixicanus*), showed similar impacts. Most affected species showed signs of recovery during the years following those outbreaks, however, Yellow-billed Magpie numbers have failed to recover to pre-WNV levels. Further, this magpie demonstrates persistent sensitivity to subsequent WNV outbreaks. These subsequent outbreaks have affected other species, but populations of those species appear to recover quickly following those outbreaks, while magpie numbers continue to decline. The range of the Yellow-billed Magpie is restricted to north-central California, and their range has constricted in recent decades with extirpation of some southern California populations. Therefore, the inability of this species to adapt to the presence of this virus is of significant conservation concern. In this chapter the author reviews the impacts of WNV on several bird species and discuss the implications for the long-term survival the Yellow-billed Magpie.

In: West Nile Virus
Editor: Marinke van Verseveld

ISBN: 978-1-53616-589-0
© 2019 Nova Science Publishers, Inc.

Chapter 1

MULTI-SPECIES, CLIMATE-DRIVEN AND LANDSCAPE-BASED CELLULAR DIFFERENCE EQUATION MODEL FOR WEST NILE VIRUS: TOWARD AN AGENT-BASED MODEL OF WEST NILE VIRUS SPREAD

Hamid Reza Nasrinpour[1], Abba Gumel[2], Marcia R. Friesen[1] and Robert D. McLeod[1],*

[1]Electrical and Computer Engineering, University of Manitoba, Winnipeg, MB, Canada
[2]School of Mathematical and Statistical Science, Arizona State University, Tempe, AZ, US

ABSTRACT

The objective of this study is to design and implement an efficient data-driven Agent-Based Model (ABM) of West Nile Virus (WNV) spread, considering highly-mobile humans with a high level of

---
* Corresponding Author's E-mail: Robert.McLeod@UManitoba.ca.

heterogeneous properties. The undeniable value of such an ABM is in simulating and assessing virtually all epidemiological scenarios and prevention strategies. This chapter proposes a Cellular Difference Equation (CDiffE) model for adoption in WNV-ABMs. The proposed CDiffE Model includes multiple species of birds and humans as hosts for the spread of WNV in Southern Manitoba. The migration patterns of different bird species, nocturnal biting activities of *Culex tarsalis* mosquitoes, daily temperature and rainfall, and land cover impact are incorporated into the model. WNV-related parameters for different bird species are estimated according to biological studies on avian viremia. The proposed CDiffE updates on an hourly step in order to act as an environment for a comprehensive agent-based model of WNV spread among peripatetic humans. In general, the model predicts mosquito distribution across the province effectively well. The mosquito population trends within the model over 15 weeks in approximately 30 communities of Manitoba has Pearson and Spearman correlation values of approximately 60% compared with the real-world mosquito trap data. The difference equations are principally much faster than commonly used differential equation models. While the whole system is designed from an agent-based modelling perspective at a cellular level, it exhibits biologically compatible behaviour at the macro-level scale. The geographical output of the current model can be considered a decision support tool for public health policymakers by providing risk maps of mosquito densities. In varying the model parameters, some theoretically verified as well as counter-intuitive findings were observed.

Keywords: agent-based model, cellular difference equation, West Nile Virus, public health policy

INTRODUCTION

West Nile Virus (WNV) was first isolated from a feverish woman in Uganda in 1937 [1]. The arrival of WNV in the American continent occurred in New York in 1999 [2]. In Canada, the mosquito infection rate and mortality of birds have been used as a proxy for WNV transmission risk. The first appearance of infected birds in Manitoba was in 2002 [3]. The highest number of human cases associated with WNV for Manitoba was reported in 2007 with 587 cases, which includes asymptomatic, neurological, non-neurological syndrome, and unclassified cases with positive test results [4]. Unfortunately, there is no specific treatment for illness resulting from WNV, and some infected humans suffer from severe symptoms such as blurred vision, meningitis, paralysis and eventually sometimes death.

In WNV transmission cycle, certain mosquitoes are vectors; birds act as amplifying hosts; and humans are incidental hosts [5–8]. A literature review on different species of mosquito vectors, bridge vectors of birds, and their traits and habitat preferences is given in the Appendix. These properties are essential knowledge when developing transmission models.

When investigating disease transmission dynamics, differential equation (DE) models are among the most noted solutions. Thomas and Urena formulated a difference equation for WNV evolution in a mosquito–bird–human community with parameters for spraying pesticide [9]. Wonham et al. developed a single-season classic susceptible-infectious-removed (SIR) DE model for WNV transmission in a bird-mosquito population [10]. Bowman et al. propose a single-season DE model of WNV transmission dynamics in a mosquito–bird–human population [11]. Cruz-Pacheco et al. [12] formulate and analyse a DE model of WNV transmission with a focus on hosts and estimating the competence of bird species. Simpson et al. [13] developed a DE model for WNV transmission with a focus on host feeding preferences using one vector species (*Cx. pipiens*) and two category of preferred and non-preferred bird hosts.

WNV transmission dynamic modelling could go further and include integrative studies where spatio-temporal co-occurrence of vectors and mobile hosts with heterogeneous population properties are modeled [14]. In this context, Agent-Based Models (ABMs) can be designed to combine features and strengths of all the DE models mentioned above into a single system. ABMs, intrinsically, can incorporate biodiversity of birds and mosquitoes, their heterogeneous contacts, and their interaction with mobile humans, without making any homogenous assumptions about the population or hard-coding any statistical rules/correlations at the system-level. Whereas exploring any additional factor in a DE model requires hard-coding of some new parameters or even re-designing the whole model at a population-level.

Agent-based modelling is a natural and intuitive way of simulating systems where individual agents (e.g., people or mosquitoes) play significant roles. In this bottom-up approach, the system contains a set of autonomous individuals, i.e., agents, interacting based on a set of rules of behaviour within an environment. From the micro-level inter-actions between agents of the same or different types, the macro-level patterns of the system emerge [15]. In WNV epidemiology, the main means of spread of the virus is the interaction cycles within different agent types (specifically birds and mosquitoes). This makes ABMs an ideal tool to investigate the epidemiology of WNV. Additionally, human behaviour and their community structure has an indisputable effect on the spread of an infectious virus (e.g., flu) [16, 17]. Yet, these factors are generally neglected in WNV models as humans are dead-end WNV hosts. Depending on the level of details implemented in an ABM, the role of each characteristic/trait of various mosquito and bird species in the WNV epidemiological system may be investigated. Also, to capture even more dynamics and phenomena, the model alterations can be done at an individual-level, if need be. More importantly, the impact of some uncertain intervention strategies and control scenarios can be effectively assessed. For example, one may wonder if building a school near a pond or a small stagnant lake (i.e., a potential hot-spot for mosquitoes) would make any difference to WNV prevalence in an area. In a WNV-ABM, it is very straightforward to discover how agents (e.g., people/mosquitoes) would respond to a change in the environmental conditions.

While the ABMs have been extensively applied in health care applications [18–21], its use in the WNV literature is rather scant. In [22], using the Repast toolkit, an ABM is constructed for an area of 165 km^2 in Cook County, Illinois, US modelled as a raster map. Three bird species of black-capped chickadee, blue jay, and American crow are considered in their work. A set of differential equations are used for virus transmission dynamics. Land cover, temperature and rainfall are used to tune the mosquito population. However, detailed equations, parameters and results are not presented. Another ABM with no human component is proposed by Bouden et al. [23] with a focus on larviciding practices. This ABM disregards the impact of land cover and considers one mosquito site per an entire municipality in southern Quebec, Canada. Their mosquito agents include two primarily bird biting species of *Cx pipiens* and *Cx restuans* with a constant biting rate during a 24-hour daily step. The total length of roads in each municipality is used to tune total mosquito population of the entire municipality. The bird agents are also classified into two groups of competent crows and the remainder with average parameters. The DE model in [10] with modifications to incorporate weather impacts are used for virus transmission dynamics. Central to all models, the lack of sufficient field data affects the model's calibration process. A review of these models and some other related ABMs can be found in [8].

Out of the WNV models reviewed, the work of Bouden et al. [23] is conceptually most similar to the proposed work. However, differences to our work are found in several key areas. For instance, the authors in [23] use differential equations applied at the level of the municipality, the two category of birds are treated as mobile roost agents, and time advances are implemented on a daily step. Our work applies differences equations, which are inherently faster than differential equations for numerical simulation. Also, our work applies a difference equation to each mosquito cell, which is a much more fine-grained implementation. Our model consists of many different bird species, yet their movement are considered at a less detailed scale. Finally, our work implements hourly time-steps, trading speed for more fine-grained outputs.

In this chapter, a data-driven Cellular Difference Equation (CDiffE) model, including a human component and multiple species of birds, is proposed to be used in ABMs for WNV propagation. As one of the goals here was to develop WNV simulation software for Manitoba, the implementation of the CDiffE is based on the data available form (or appropriate for) this region. Yet, the model design is more general and applicable to other areas. Compared to difference equation models, differential equation models have been applied more often in both WNV and ABM literature [8], and this chapter demonstrates that difference equation models offer a valuable approach to optimizing the trade-off between a model's computational complexity and its inherent ability to consider multiple agent types at very fine-grained and individual profile levels. Difference equations are inherently faster for numerical computations, as they do not require a slow ordinary differential equation (ODE) solver to be triggered in each iteration of the algorithm. That is vital for ABMs as they generally suffer from computational complexities, as such, difference equations fit better within their realm. The proposed difference equation model is cellular as it requires the spatial input domain to be rasterized. The model considers landscape features, temperature and rainfall, circadian changes in mosquito behaviour, weekly bird migration patterns, and bird characteristics by species. The model output is validated against carbon dioxide baited trap data in terms of Pearson and Spearman correlations.

METHODS

In this section, the proposed cellular model is described. The region of study (i.e., Manitoba) is modeled as a grid map where each cell represents a 5 km x 5 km mosquito site (Figure 1). Each mosquito site (or cell) has its own unique landscape features and is assigned to a rural municipality's weather station. There are around 6,000 mosquito sites covering the scope of the model in Southern Manitoba. The main mosquito species considered in the model is *Cx. tarsalis*. Around 150 different species of bird, including local and migratory birds known to be infected with WNV, are present in Manitoba in summer. The data about the location and population count of these different bird species are collected [24]. These locations are referred to as bird roosts. A roost is where birds spend their night. Unlike the mosquito sites, sizes of different roosting sites are different and may be shared by more than one bird species at a time. In the model, due to differences of various bird species (such as different virus competence indices), a bird roost is considered for every single species of bird located at the same roosting site. From an ABM perspective, mosquito sites and bird roosts are agents in the model.

Using the BAM (Boreal Avian Modelling) [25] estimation method in [24], there are over 70,000 bird roosts in the model. Each mosquito site is associated with a number of bird roosts depending on the size and coordinates of the roost, and the home range of the bird. On average, each mosquito site is covered by (and consequently linked to) 30 bird roosts.

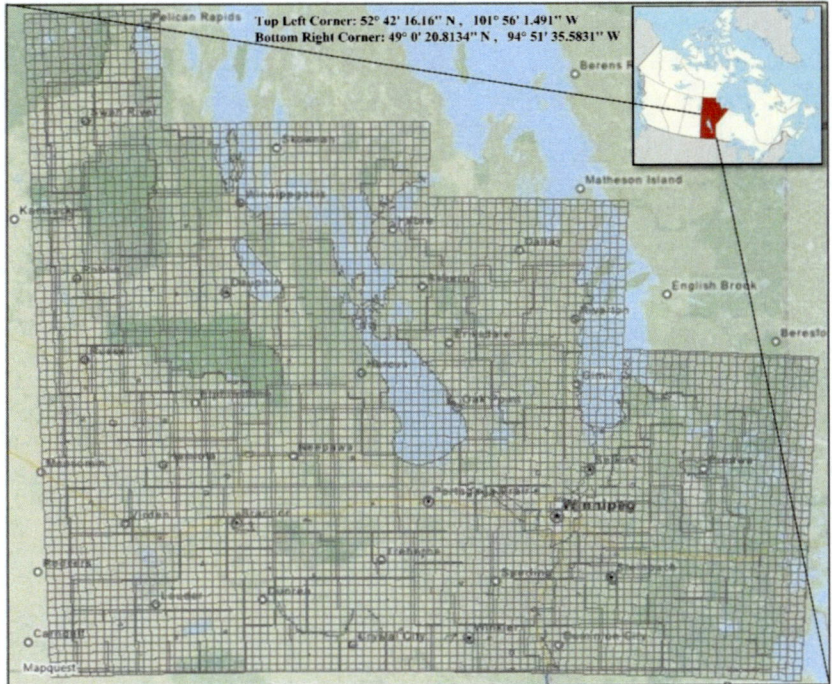

Figure 1. Southern Manitoba map showing the mosquito grid as an overlay.

Difference Equation Model Basis

An instance of the proposed difference equation model is cloned in each mosquito cell (site). In every hourly time-step, the equations update for all the active mosquito sites. The dynamics of all agents (mosquito sites, bird roosts, and humans) update based on the proposed set of difference equations, which consider the interactions of the following key parameters: Daily mean Temperature, T, Daily Rainfall, R, and the Landscape descriptor, L. The proposed difference equation model is built upon the differential equation model of Wonham et al. [10] using the approach in Lewis et al.

[26] with further extensions to include humans, various birds species, and impact of temperature, rainfall, and landscape features (so-called land use/cover).

The core of the proposed difference equation model has some fundamental changes compared to Lewis et al.'s [26]. A key change is that the equations are modified to include multiple bird species, making the contact rate and the probability of transmission of virus from an infectious mosquito to a bird different for various bird species. Also, some other extensions are incorporated to include human components and the impact of changes in the population of birds due to migration. The core of the proposed difference equation model is as follows, with the parameter definitions in Table 1.

Mosquito Equations:

$$M_a(t+1) = r\,(1-\mu_a)\bigl(M_s(t)+M_i(t)\bigr) + (1-\mu_a)(1-\gamma)M_a(t) \tag{1}$$

$$M_s(t+1) = (1-\mu_m)(1-\beta_m)^{e_m(t)}\,M_s(t) + (1-\mu_m)\,\gamma\,M_a(t) \tag{2}$$

$$M_i(t+1) = (1-\mu_m)\bigl(1-(1-\beta_m)^{e_m(t)}\bigr)M_s(t) + (1-\mu_m)M_i(t) \tag{3}$$

where

$$e_m(t) = \frac{\sum_j b^j B_i^j(t)}{H_t(t)+\sum_j B_t^j(t)} \tag{4}$$

Bird Equations:

$$B_s^j(t+1) = \left[(1-\beta_b^j)^{e_b^j(t)} B_s^j(t)\right]\eta^j(t_w) + B_m^j(t_w) \tag{5}$$

$$B_i^j(t+1) = \left[(1-\delta^j)\left(1-(1-\beta_b^j)^{e_b^j(t)}\right)B_s^j(t) + (1-\delta^j)(1-\zeta_b^j)B_i^j(t)\right]\eta^j(t_w) \quad (6)$$

$$B_r^j(t+1) = \left[\zeta_b^j B_i^j(t) + B_r^j(t)\right]\eta^j(t_w) \quad (7)$$

where

$$e_b^j(t) = \frac{b^j M_i(t)}{H_t(t) + \sum_j B_t^j(t)} \quad (8)$$

$$B_m^j(t_w) = \begin{cases} B_w^j(t_w) - B_t^j(t_w) & ; B_w^j(t_w) > B_t^j(t_w) \\ 0 & ; otherwise \end{cases} \quad (9)$$

$$\eta^j(t_w) = \begin{cases} 1 & ; B_w^j(t_w) > B_t^j(t_w) \\ \frac{B_w^j(t_w)}{B_t^j(t_w)} & ; otherwise \end{cases} \quad (10)$$

Human Equations:

$$H_s(t+1) = (1-\beta_h)^{e_h(t)} H_s(t) \quad (11)$$

$$H_i(t+1) = \left(1-(1-\beta_h)^{e_h(t)}\right)H_s(t) + (1-\zeta_h)H_i(t) \quad (12)$$

$$H_r(t+1) = \zeta_h H_i(t) + H_r(t) \quad (13)$$

where

$$e_h(t) = \frac{b_h M_i(t)}{H_t(t) + \sum_j B_t^j(t)} \quad (14)$$

is the expected number of times a human is bitten by an infectious mosquito at the time-step t. Similarly, $e_b^j(t)$ is the expected number of times a bird of specie j is bitten by an infectious mosquito, and $e_m(t)$ is the expected number of times a mosquito bites an infectious bird. Also, the two parameters of $B_m^j(t_w)$ and $\eta^j(t_w)$ keep track of changes in the population of birds of species j in week t_w according to the real weekly population data (B_w).

Table 1. General Notations

	Mosquito	Birds	Human
State variables			
Aquatic stage (including eggs and larvae)	M_a		
Susceptible (adult)	M_s	B_s	H_s
Infectious (adult)	M_i	B_i	H_i
Recovered (adult)		B_r	H_r
Total adults		B_t	H_t
Core parameters			
Reproduction (combining egg laying and larval hatching)	r		
Maturation probability (i.e., developing into adult mosquitoes)	γ		
Natural death probability (for aquatic and adult mosquitoes)	μ_a, μ_m		
Probability of death due to infection (for birds)		δ	
Probability of virus transmission to	β_m	β_b	β_h
Mosquito biting on host (no of bites per mosquito per time step)		B	b_h
Probability of recovery from virus		ζ_b	ζ_h
Virus incubation probability	k_m		
Bird migration parameters			
Weekly real-world count of population		B_w	
Number of (weekly) immigrant birds		B_m	
Proportion of (weekly) emigrant birds		η	
Dynamic parameters			
Mean daily positive Temperature (in Celsius)	T		
Daily Rainfall (in mm)	R		
Mean correlation between mosquito land cover and virus	L		
Daylight hours	D		
Other variables/parameters			
Species index (for birds)		j	
Normalized host competency index (for birds)		c	
Average hourly probability of biting on hosts		$\bar{b}$	$\bar{b}$
Expected number of contacts with an infectious agent	e_m	e_b	e_h
Hourly time-step	t	t	t
Weekly time-step	t_w	t_w	t_w
Ratio of mosquito biting activities between nights and days	$\omega > 1$		
Ratio of biting on birds to biting on humans	$\lambda > 1$		
Importance of landscape features for mosquito habitat	w_L		

Therefore at the beginning of each week, the total number of each bird species $B_t^j(t_w)$ will match the real-world count of bird species $B_w^j(t_w)$ that are present during the week (t_w). A value of less than one for η implies the real-world estimated population is less than the number of bird species within the simulation. As such, a proportion of birds from all compartments are assumed to leave the model scope (e.g., due to migration). Whereas when η is greater than one, (immigrant) birds are added to the susceptible compartment. As noted in Table 1, the variables t and t_w indicate time-steps whereas the subscript t in B_t and H_t denotes the total value of its associated state variable (i.e., B for bird population and H for human population).

Weather and Landscape Impacts

The core difference equation model is further modified to take into account the impacts of daily weather (i.e., T and R) variations and landscape features (L). As a result, reproduction per time-unit, hourly maturation (or development) probability, and hourly probability of natural death of aquatic and adult mosquitoes in mosquito dynamics equations update on a daily basis according to the weather functions proposed in [27]. The mosquitoes biting rate (i.e., number per unit of time) is also a function of temperature and host preference, and is accounted for in the model. The parameters of the weather functions from [27] are then tuned to the weather and mosquito surveillance data in Southern Manitoba. This calibration procedure is explained in a later section.

The reproduction parameter also depends on the different classes of land use/cover present in a mosquito site/cell (i.e., the parameter L). For each mosquito site, the proportional area of each land cover class is known. According to the Manitoba Land Initiative [28], there are 18 known and one unknown class of land cover identified in our land cover/use dataset. The landscape descriptor, L, evaluates the habitat suitability of a mosquito cell based on the land cover types present in the cell. The impact of this parameter (L) on mosquito reproduction is controlled by another weight parameter, denoted as w_L. The exact mathematical relation of all these parameters to the proposed core Difference Equation (DiffE) model can be found in the Appendix.

Multiple Bird Species and Rates

The model assumes that the transmission probability from an infected mosquito bite to a bird is 100% [29]. Second, there is no infected bird compartment in our proposed difference equation model, but only the infectious bird compartment. This means a bird is marked as infectious only if the infected bird has the competency to transmit the virus to another mosquito vector. Otherwise, the infected bird remains a susceptible bird in the model.

Reservoir competence indices of an infected bird describe the relative proportion of vector mosquitoes that become infectious after feeding on such a bird [29, 30]. Host competence indices are calculated from species viremia level reported in [29–40]. Indices are then normalized to be between zero and one. These indices help estimate the probability of transmission between bird and mosquito, given the contact rate. The exact reasoning and formula to derive host competence indices can be found in [30]. Normalized host competence indices for some of the birds' species can be found in the Appendix.

It is notable that a natural death is not possible for birds as the model is seasonal (i.e., it runs only for one spring and summer per simulation year). However, the data-driven weekly variations in bird population is accounted for in the proposed CDiffE model. Where the experimental studies are available for a species, death (due to infection) and recovery rates are estimated, and the corresponding probabilities are then calculated. Where the experimental data are missing for a species, estimation of death and recovery rates for each species are estimated from average values of other species in the same family or order where data is available. Exact mathematical details and the estimated daily rates and hourly probabilities for a number of bird species can be found in the Appendix.

Moreover, the majority of host-seeking activities of *Culex* mosquito occurs at nights [41, 42], and this is reflected in the average hourly biting probability. It is notable that the biting rate (i.e., the number of bites made per mosquito per time step) on humans is much lower than the birds' biting rate. More discussion on the biting rates and probabilities as well as the details of modelling mosquito nocturnal activities can be found in the Appendix.

Avian Flow

In WNV epidemiology, the movement of birds is not as critical to the model as their roosting activities [43, 44]. The reason is that the majority of birds get bitten and infected while they roost. As such, spotting a bird roost is more influential than modelling bird (long-distance) movement patterns. Yet, short flights to surrounding areas in search of food is the primary way of spreading the infection. Generally, the breeding seasons of the birds in the system are within the span of simulation time (i.e., spring/summer). Given this and the tendency to simplify the computational complexity of the avian flow, birds were assumed to remain close to their nesting locations at nights, and to fly around during the day within their home-range but still close to their nests. Therefore, the value of total number of birds per each mosquito cell is different depending on the hour of the day.

A typical bird roost is covered by a number of mosquito site agents. After each time-step, some birds of a roost may become infectious as a result of contact with different mosquito (site) agents. Therefore, at the beginning of the next step, there is a probability that a bird that became infectious from the mosquito site X would spread the infection to the mosquito site Y, as long as both mosquito sites X and Y reside within the home range of the bird. Basically at each time-step, the total population of birds of a roost is split proportionally among all the mosquito sites covered by the birds, assuming a homogenous and well-mixed population of bird agents.

Moreover, unlike the classical assumption of difference and differential equation models where every vector (mosquito) could bite and infect every host (birds), it is considered that only a certain proportion of mosquitoes in a site could bite birds of a certain roost provided that the roost is *not* completely covered by the mosquito site.

Each species of bird has different home ranges and may fly up to a certain maximum distance for their food seeking activities. While the average number of birds present in the simulation per mosquito cells can be calculated, the actual number of birds per each mosquito cell is quite different at each hour. The weekly trends of average number of birds per mosquito cell is given in Figure 2. At the beginning of the simulation, the figure is over 11,000. It then goes up with a few fluctuations during the spring and summer until the last weeks of simulations where it gradually decreases to an approximate value of 8,000.

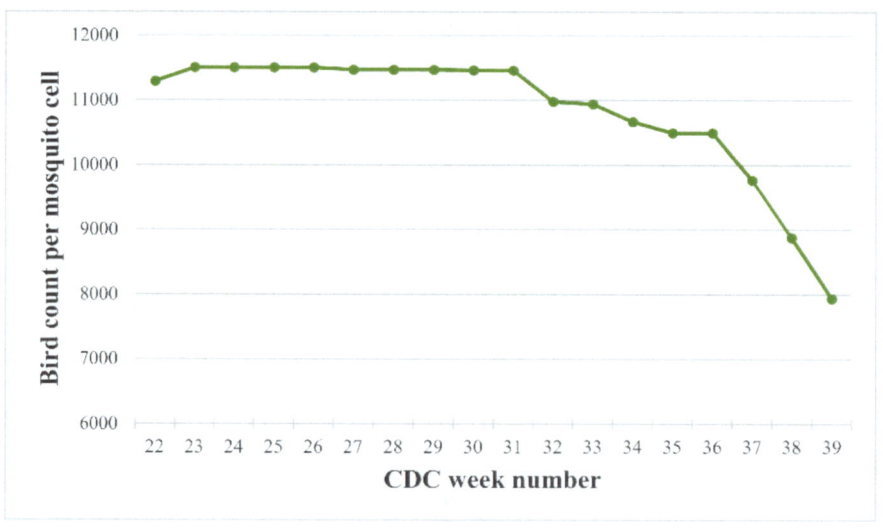

Figure 2. Weekly trends of average number of birds per mosquito cell.

PARAMETER CALIBRATION AND MODEL VALIDATION

Parameter calibration is achieved by comparing the total mosquito count in the model against the Centers for Disease Control (CDC) carbon dioxide baited trap data [4]. The trap data are the number of mosquitoes per collection night, which can be inferred as the average weekly count of total mosquitoes. These data were available from the CDC week 22 to CDC week 36 (a total of 15 weeks) for approximately 30 communities in Manitoba from 2004 to 2014 [4]. The data from 2004 to 2013 are used as training data for calibration and tuning purposes, and the data from 2014 is then used for validation as the test data.

In the model, the count of total adult mosquitoes from all mosquito sites of each community is recorded only at mid-night to avoid overestimating the nightly population counts. This is conceptually similar to having mosquito traps run for an hour each night. This figure is then divided by the number of days in a week and the total area of mosquito sites in each community, so that the average nightly count/density per one km^2 is obtained for each community each week. For the calibration purposes, the output for each simulated year is defined as a matrix of these average weekly mosquito counts. The matrix has around 30 rows (for communities) and 15 columns (for weeks). The correlation between this simulation output matrix and the trap data matrix are then calculated for each year. The average correlation between simulation output and trap data for years 2004 to 2013 is used as a fitness function in the optimization algorithm. While the optimization algorithm could be any metaheuristic search algorithm, we employed the Grouped Bees Algorithm [45] in conjunction with the OptQuest optimization engine [46].

The correlation between the simulation output and the trap data indicates how well the model predicts weekly trends of mosquito population counts in different locations/communities. It also captures variations in mosquito distributions over different locations/communities in a certain week. Unfortunately, the ratio of the number of captured mosquito to the actual population of mosquito varies by region and month [60]. Based on the experiments in [60], it may be inferred that a captured *Culex tarsalis* mosquito represents around 300 mosquitoes over one km^2 in August. Consequently, a simplifying assumption was made that the scaling factor of 300 remains the same in the entire simulation time. More discussion on the calibration challenges can be found in the Appendix.

RESULTS AND DISCUSSION

Calibration Results

The calibration process results in acceptable trends of mosquito population dynamics for both test and training data. The calibration procedure can also end up with different sets of solutions, depending on how the weights and penalties are set in the fitness function. Furthermore, surprisingly, the weight (w_L) of landscape factor (L) on mosquito habitat was set at a relatively low (and positive) value. A discussion on this parameter is given in the Appendix.

Here, the solutions for three general cases of correlation-oriented, population-oriented, and balanced-approach are presented as examples. Three evaluation metrics of Spearman's rank-order correlation, Pearson correlation and logarithmic-scale population ratio for each solution is given in Table 2, where the logarithmic-scale population ratio is defined as

$$\text{Pop. Ratio} = \frac{\ln(P_s)}{\ln(P_t \times 300)}$$

where P_t is the total number of weekly captured mosquitoes from the trap data for each year and P_s is the sum of average weekly density of mosquitoes per one km² in selected communities (i.e., corresponding to the trap data communities) generated by the simulation for each year.

According to Table 2, the correlation-oriented solutions have higher correlations (both Spearman and Pearson) with an average of approximately 60% in all years (including both training and test years). The Population-oriented solutions have the lowest correlation values but the highest population ratio with an average of approximately 73% in all years. The balanced-approach solutions fall in between with an average of approximately 52% correlation and 68% population ratio. A correlation value of around 60% for weekly variations over various regions may not be considered a high value. However, in a WNV study on birds infection rates in Ontario, Canada [47], the Pearson correlation between observed and predicted values for monthly variations in Ontario (i.e., only a single location) fall between 60% to 63% for training and test data using an artificial neural network technique. It is notable that neural networks are theorized to be universal approximators with acceptable accuracy.

Table 2. Calibration results; for three different sets of solutions, values of correlation between trap data and simulation output for training and test years, as well as ratio of mosquito population in simulations to trap data are reported

Training years	Correlation-oriented			Population-oriented			Balanced-approach		
	Pearson	Spearman	Pop. Ratio	Pearson	Spearman	Pop. Ratio	Pearson	Spearman	Pop. Ratio
2004	62%	60%	54%	76%	65%	65%	73%	66%	61%
2005	90%	71%	54%	68%	65%	70%	86%	67%	61%
2006	61%	39%	64%	22%	22%	79%	38%	29%	72%
2007	44%	52%	53%	4%	15%	70%	24%	29%	62%
2008	86%	70%	53%	63%	69%	64%	78%	70%	60%
2009	18%	32%	64%	23%	28%	76%	23%	27%	70%
2010	77%	71%	63%	28%	56%	78%	55%	63%	69%
2011	79%	58%	63%	54%	55%	75%	66%	56%	70%
2012	73%	52%	62%	39%	42%	76%	56%	45%	69%
2013	35%	45%	66%	12%	50%	79%	28%	43%	72%
Average	62%	55%	59%	39%	47%	73%	53%	50%	68%
Test year									
2014	73%	64%	59%	51%	61%	74%	62%	60%	68%

Although direct numerical comparison between the two models is not necessarily meaningful, there are conceptual links between the two. Generally, high number of mosquitoes is correlated with high number of infection in both mosquitoes and birds, assuming the presence of the virus. However, this should not be taken to imply that neural networks cannot achieve greater predictive power for WNV epidemiology. The value of proposed CDiffE model, and in particular agent-based modelling, in this context is in construction of a virtual simulation framework in order to assess many different influential factors in WNV epidemiology before putting them in practice. Such simulators will help to elucidate the underlying mechanism of WNV propagation. Generally transparent simulation methods such as ABM provide insight into the subject of study in comparison with the black box approach offered by soft computing techniques such as neural networks. Further discussion of the table is presented later.

Model Validation

Overall, according to Table 2, the model has an acceptable predictive power of approximately 60% in terms of correlation between the trap data and simulation output for mosquito population dynamics. To provide a better visual insight into these quantities, two more figures are presented. First, Figure 3 compares the scaled weekly trend of total trapped mosquitoes from the data against the weekly mosquito densities generated by simulation using the balanced-approach solution. The figure is depicted for all the years from 2004 to 2014. In most years the trends of mosquito population dynamics in simulation output is close to the total number of mosquitoes collected weekly in Manitoba traps.

The worst performances are for years 2009 and 2007. 2007 is when the highest number of WNV human cases and captured mosquito counts were observed in Manitoba. For some reasons, in 2007, a primary peak of mosquito (host-seeking) activity was observed in week 26 whereas the simulation does not capture any unusual increases in mosquito population. This might be due to unexpected changes in bird populations. In current simulations, bird populations are assumed to have the same migration patterns and roosting locations in all the simulated years. It is notable to mention that the trap data provides information on female host-seeking mosquitoes, not actually the count for the entire mosquito population. This means if there are not many hosts to feed on, there may not be many host-seeking mosquitoes, despite having a highly mosquito-populated area. On the other hand, if there are no real available hosts, then the traps, as they mimic a possible host by releasing CO_2, may even capture more mosquitoes.

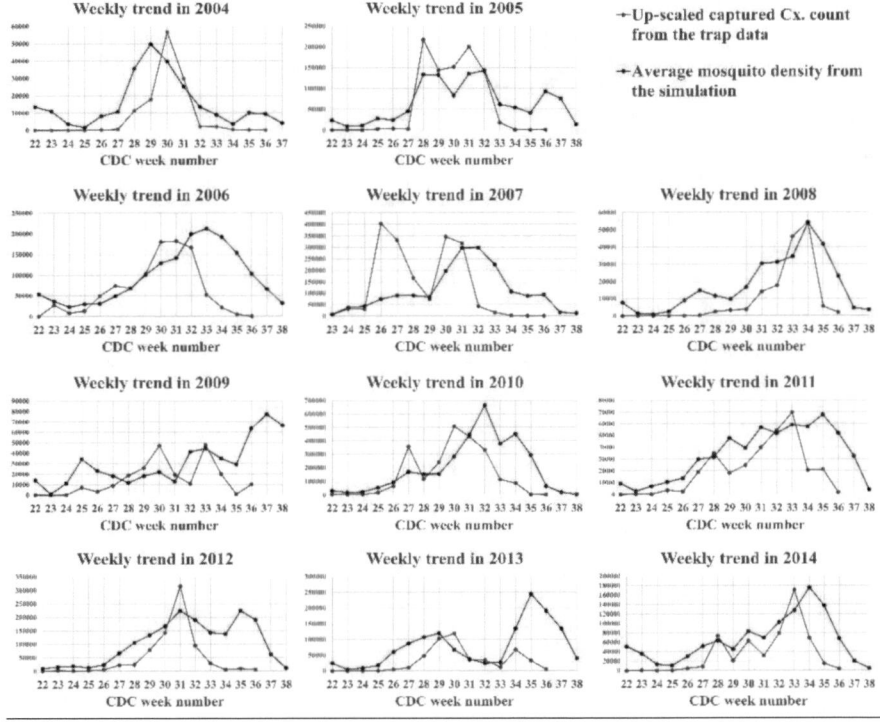

Figure 3. Weekly trends of sum of scaled trap data versus simulation's weekly mosquito densities for 2004 to 2014.

Generally, when rain of around 10 mm to 25 mm with temperature of occasionally 20°C (or slightly above it) occurs in the same week, the model fails to flush a sufficient number of larvae. Therefore, we often observe a visible increase (or maybe a jump depending on temperature) in the number of mosquitoes in the model, whereas a drop or only a slight increase is expected. The impacts were strong enough in some years (e.g., 2009 and 2013) to significantly drop the correlation values. Examples of such co-incident events include week 32 in 2007, weeks 25 and 32 in 2009, and weeks 26 and 34 in 2013.

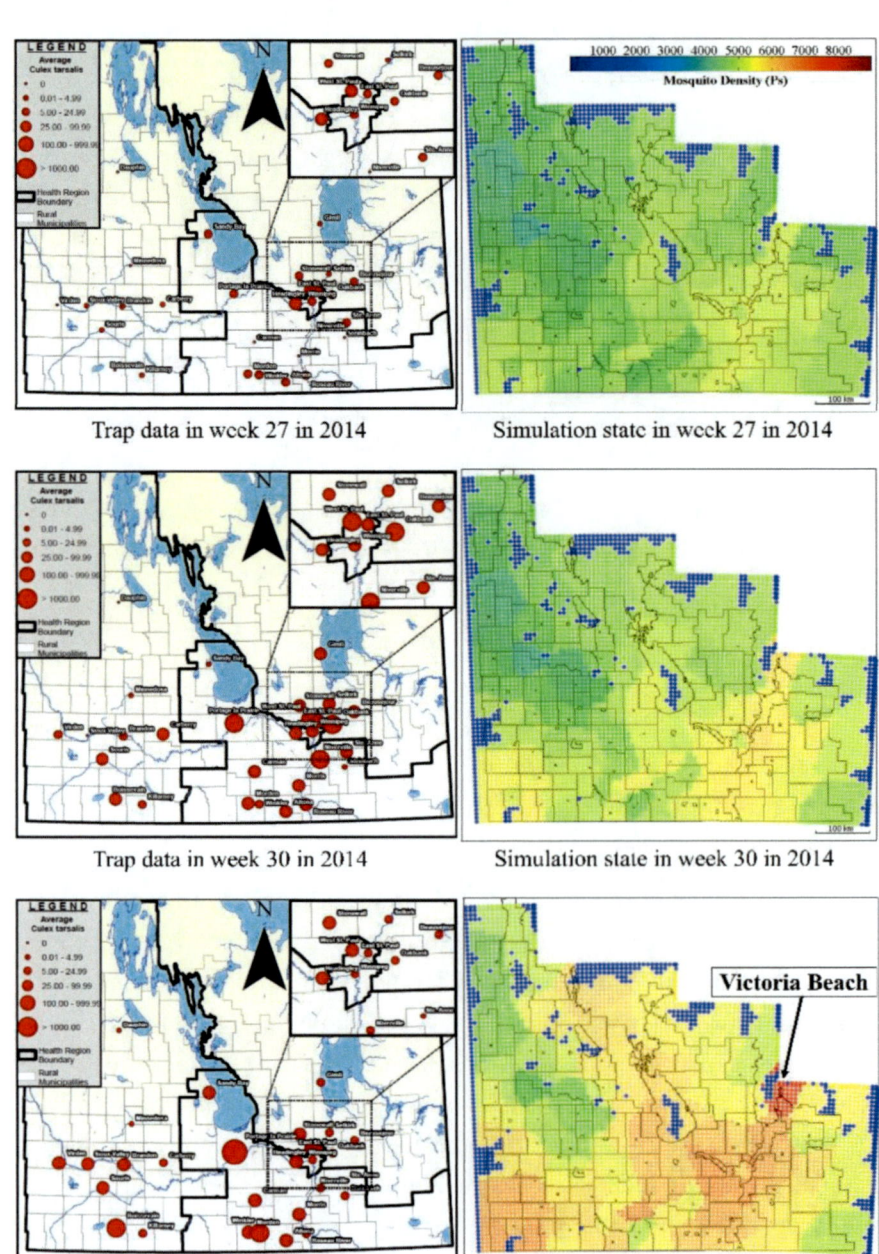

Source: Manitoba Health [4].

Figure 4. Side-by-side comparison of weekly distribution of mosquitoes across the province according to the trap data and simulation.

It can be seen, in general, in the last weeks of simulations, the system has more mosquitoes than the trap data suggests. This is most likely due to diapause [48], when mosquitoes become dormant towards the fall based on the changing daylight length. Put differently, in those relatively cool weeks, there are still mosquitoes in the area, but they are not active enough to get captured at the traps. Incorporating the diapause process would be particularly important to obtain a better fit of mosquito population, if the simulation had to capture whole year dynamics. Moreover, always in week 22, the simulation has more mosquitoes than the trap data, which likely is because of the initial simulation conditions. For further visual comparison, Figure 4 compares the mosquito geographic distribution in a number of weeks between the simulation and trap data in Manitoba. For each week, in Figure 4, two images are shown: (1) trap data of the week on left [4], (2) mosquito density generated by the simulation during the same week on right. The simulation screenshots for this experiment were taken while the simulation was running for the test year of 2014. It is immediately clear from the screenshots in Figure 4 that the model output correctly identifies the mosquito patterns at the province-scale. Figure 4 also suggests the Victoria beach area could be a potential hot spot for mosquito activities; however, no mosquito trap is installed there to judge this conjecture. This must be mainly due to the generally warm weather conditions of this area over a long period of time. In fact, in most years in our dataset, the vicinity of the Victoria beach was one of the hottest areas in the province from the middle of July until the first weeks of September. Further discussion on this experiment is given in the Appendix.

Infectious Propagation

Simulations on infection propagation demonstrated that the birds are the main factors for spreading WNV to distant areas. As an example, the test year of 2014 was selected as the input for the simulation of this section. A total of half a percent (0.005) of mosquito population was set to be infectious by infecting half of the population of one percent of mosquito cells/sites.

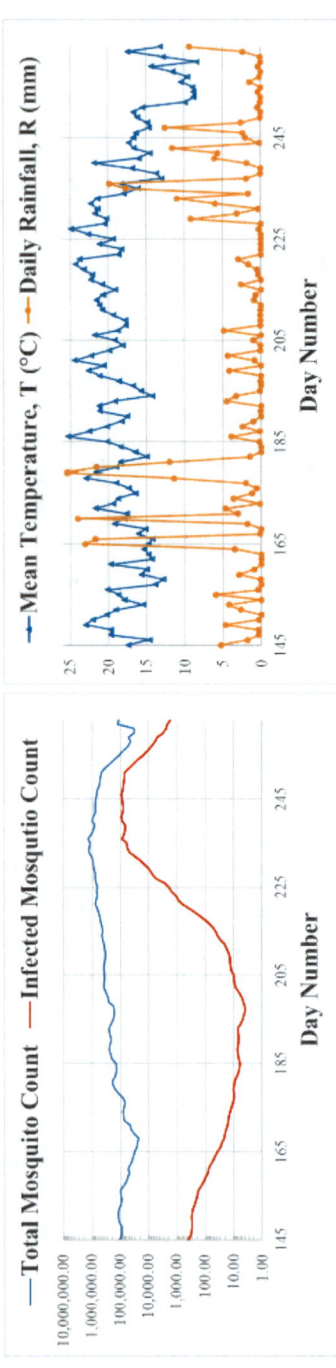

Figure 5. Left: The number of total adult and infected adult mosquitoes in a logarithmic-scale; Right: Daily values of mean Temperature (°C) and mean Rainfall (mm).

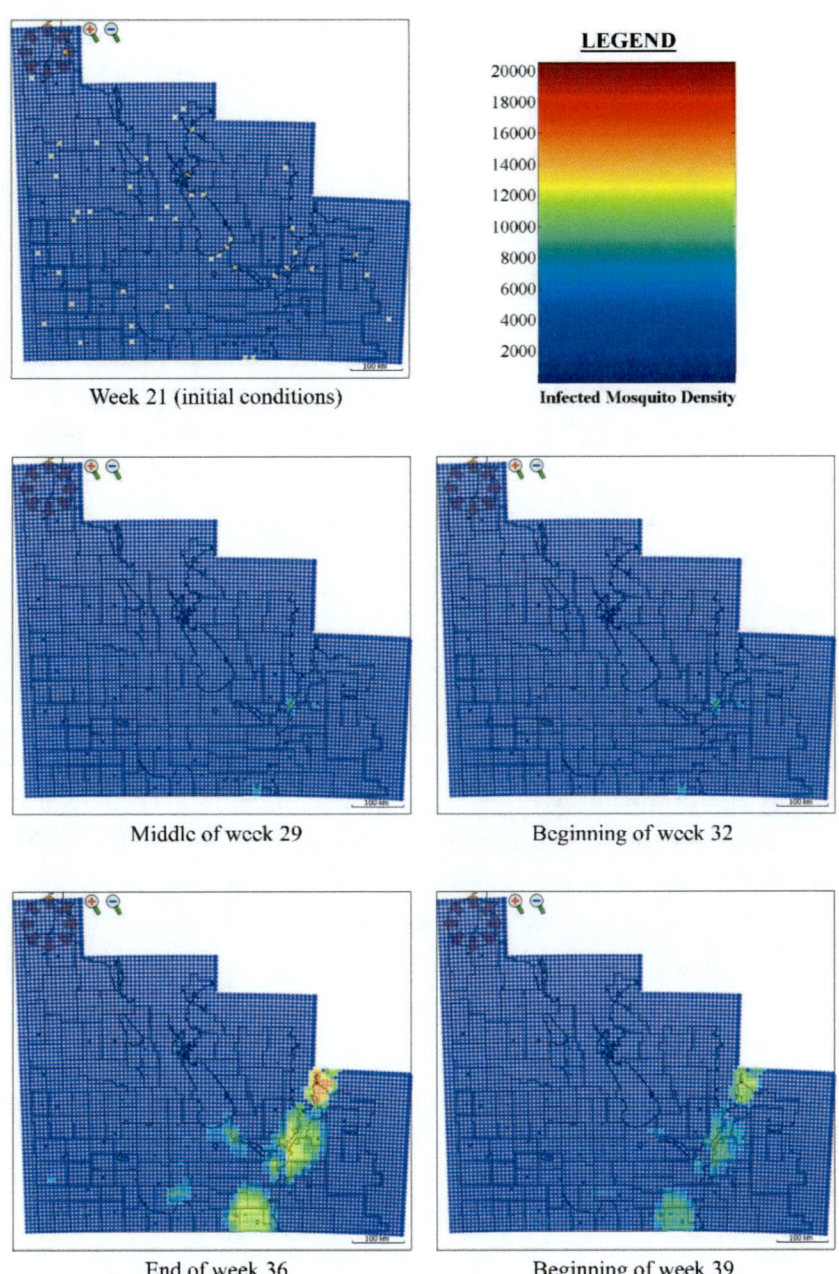

Figure 6. The distribution of infected mosquitoes across the province in a number of weeks for an arbitrary input climate.

The number of initially infected mosquitoes is high enough to initially infect a few of birds before those mosquitoes die out. Therefore, it is quite reasonable to assume some competent birds at those initially infected mosquito sites are infectious until they either recover or die.

Figure 5 shows variation of daily rainfall, temperature, and the number of total mosquitoes and infected ones for this simulation in a logarithmic-scale. Figure 6 illustrates the spread of the infection across the province over a number of weeks. Week 21 in Figure 6 shows the initial location of infected mosquito sites in a lime color. These mosquitoes infect some birds around them. By the middle of week 29 (i.e., day no. 194), the majority of the infected mosquitoes die out as the map is entirely blue, but there still exist some infectious birds. Beginning the week 32, the infection in mosquitoes has begun emerging mostly in the areas close to the initially infected mosquito sites as these areas have the highest number of infectious birds, and they may still have infected mosquitoes. The infectious birds from these areas could fly over other mosquito sites and spread WNV to them. During the weeks 34-35, a rather sharp increase occurs in the population of mosquitoes in mosquito-favored areas, such as the Victoria Beach on top right of the map. Therefore, these highly mosquito-populated sites have a relatively high probability of biting an infectious bird, even though there were *not* any infectious birds/mosquitoes, initially. Later on, at the beginning of week 39, the mosquitoes activities (and consequently the number of infected mosquitoes) is reduced everywhere due to changes in weather conditions. Figure 6 confirms the avian flow of the system is in a significant factor in WNV propagation to other locations.

Sensitivity Report

The primary findings of the Sensitivity Analysis were that the output of the CDiffE is sensitive to all the key inputs (i.e., temperature, rainfall, and land cover factor). Increasing the value of w_L (i.e., Landscape impact) yields an increase in the average Pearson correlation between the trap data and simulation output. Increases in daily temperature and rainfall values up to some thresholds also increase mosquito infection rates, although, temperature has a more influential impact.

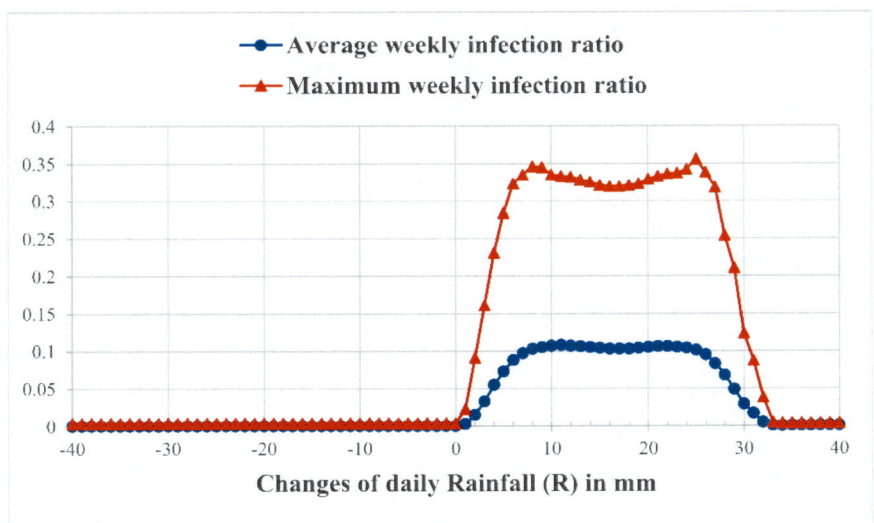

Figure 7. Variations of weekly infection ratio, being averaged for 2003 to 2014, with respect to changes in the daily value of Rainfall (R).

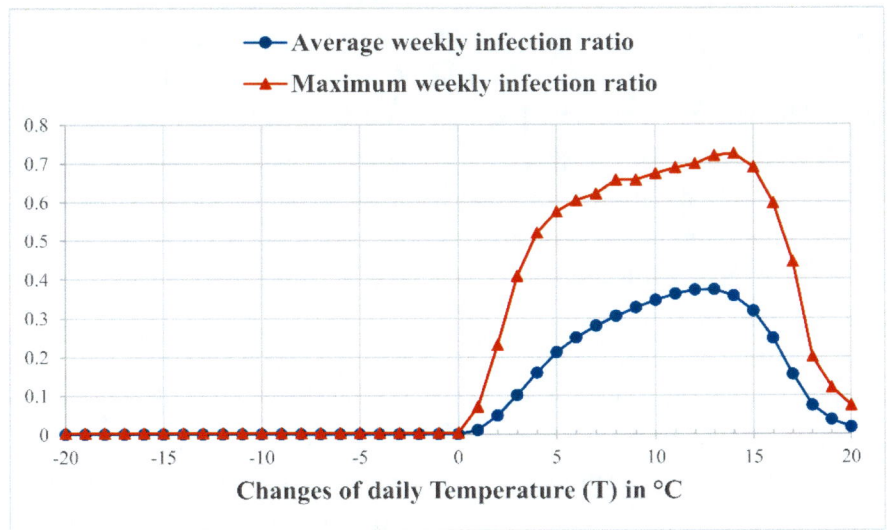

Figure 8. Variations of weekly infection ratio, being averaged for 2003 to 2014, with respect to changes in the daily value of mean Temperature (T).

For the brevity, changes to the value of w_L is not discussed here, but can be found in the Appendix. In addition to the three evaluation metrics of mosquito population, a weekly infection ratio is calculated for mosquitoes during the simulations. The weekly infection ratio can be used to decide whether an input scenario results in an outbreak depending on the competence-level of target hosts. Figure 7 and Figure 8 demonstrate changes of the 'total average' and 'average of yearly maxima' of weekly infection ratios with respect to changes in daily values of mean temperature and rainfall for all the years from 2003 to 2014. For each input value of the horizontal axes in Figure 7 and Figure 8, the values of Rainfall and Temperature for all days were changed accordingly. For example, an input value of -10 mm in Figure 7 means 10 mm is subtracted from the rainfall values of all simulated days (and truncated at zero). Similarly a value of 10°C on the horizontal axis in Figure 8 means 10°C is added to the mean daily temperature of all simulated days. The temperature value is also truncated at zero (i.e., it never has a negative value).

Both maximum and average weekly infection ratios have similar trends as shown in Figure 7 and Figure 8. Overall, the two plots indicate the model is extremely sensitive to weather conditions as expected.

The desired level and frequency of rainfall for mosquitoes is controversial [14, 49, 50]. An in depth discussion on the impacts of precipitation needs to address the difference in the mosquito species across the different studies. However, it is generally safe to assume that wet weather conditions amplify the occurrence of mosquito-borne diseases [51]. According to Figure 6, if the amount of daily rainfall for each day increases by 2 to 32 mm, a visible increase occurs in weekly infection ratios, compared to a change of zero mm in daily rainfalls. This change has three phases of a sharp positive increase, followed by a relatively constant interval, and a sharp decrease. The double-sided effect of rainfall can be explained through mosquito habitat preferences for breeding and a larvae flushing effect of heavy rainfalls. This trend verifies the fact that small increases in rainfall generally create more stagnant water for mosquitoes to lay eggs, whereas heavy rainfall flushes and kills them [52]. The other interesting and less intuitive phenomenon was slight changes of infection ratios for negative values of the horizontal axis (i.e., rainfall changes) in Figure 7. While it may not be visible in the plot-scale of Figure 7, the rainfall change of -40 to -15 mm resulted in a slightly higher infection ratio, compared to rainfall changes of -15 to 0 mm. This means the mosquitoes may do slightly better in drought conditions compared to normal rainfall conditions. The impact on mosquitoes' predators and victims may be the reason that mosquitoes do slightly better in drought even though low rainfall may not have created new breeding locations for mosquitoes. In fact, at first glance, drought reduces the necessary water for mosquito breeding, but further investigation provides facts to reinforce a drought hypothesis in favor of mosquito habitat [51, 53, 54].

By comparing the amplitude of infection ratio changes in Figure 7 and Figure 8, it is evident that mosquito dynamics are considerably more sensitive to temperature than precipitation. This is confirmed by biological studies as the temperature affects more mosquito conditions such as reproduction rate, biting rate and even WNV incubation period [14, 49, 52, 55–61]. The general trend of the plot of Figure 8 indicates increasing the mean daily temperature generally increases the infection ratio at different rates up to a high temperature where mosquitoes begin to die out due to extremely hot temperatures. Figure 8 suggests if the mean temperature of every day increases to over 20°C the death rate of mosquitoes would be so high that infection ratio would probably decline.

CONCLUSION

The primary contribution of this chapter toward an enhanced understanding of WNV transmission is the proposal and validation of a comprehensive and efficient cellular difference equation (CDiffE) structure for modelling WNV dynamics for adoption in data-driven WNV-ABMs. Differential Equations or other aggregative approaches do not have the capacity to capture WNV at a fine-grained scale. Straight ABMs are too expensive to model virus transmissions at the agent-levels (i.e., triggering rules per every single mosquito). In a hybrid ABM-based approach, difference equations should be exploited as opposed to differential equations. In addition, a cellular map, as opposed to polygon-shaped boundaries [23] or virtual networks [62], makes it easy to effectively analyze spatial aspects of WNV such as human mobility. This chapter showed how hybrid methods can effectively capture the spatio-temporal dynamics with an acceptable accuracy and computational cost.

This chapter focussed on including as many WNV factors related to mosquito population dynamics as possible. The parameters of the difference equation are temperature- and rainfall-driven during the mosquito season. The impacts of landscape features (i.e., land cover) are included in the equations. Multiple species of local and migratory birds with their weekly migration patterns are considered as the amplifying hosts in the equations. Human agents as the dead-end hosts are included in the set of proposed equations. The twilight times are employed to set the mosquito biting rates. These parameters, specific to southern Manitoba [24], are fed into the simulations for numerical analyses. The parameters regarding the mosquito population development are calibrated based on the trap data available from the Manitoba government. For over 150 bird species, WNV-related parameters, such as competence indices and recovery rates (and probabilities), are estimated based on viremia studies.

As part of model validation, variation of mosquito densities over 15 weeks during the spring and summer for the years 2004 to 2014 is compared against the simulation outputs. Generally, simulations produce close trends of mosquito population to the actual mosquito population. The system identifies the patterns of mosquito density in approximately 30 communities over 15 weeks, relatively well.

A key contribution of the chapter is that given a set of input climate data, the system could be used as a tool to detect whether the mosquito population would be increasing, decreasing or staying constant, assuming no unexpected changes to bird conditions and land cover structures. The model output can be used as risk maps for guiding practitioners and public health authorities in Manitoba.

Key findings from the simulations suggest the vicinity of Victoria Beach in Manitoba has a relatively high potential to be a home-base for *Culex* mosquitoes. Installing mosquito traps in its proximity may be an option for the local health authorities, considering the operational expenses. The simulations predict that global warming has a drastic impact on mosquito population if no larviciding program is in effect. Moreover, the simulations exhibit biologically compatible behaviour for extreme weather conditions such as drought where mosquitoes could do relatively well in retaining their population.

The proposed CDiffE model on its own can be seen as a cellular agent-based model. Direct applications to other diseases are possible, in that the CDiffE architecture with some modifications can be utilized to describe dynamics of other mosquito-borne diseases such as Zika and dengue in other geographical areas with known historical data.

FUTURE RESEARCH AND LIMITATIONS

Certainly more simulations can be set up to further investigate the impact of many other parameters, such as bird migration patterns, their competence indices and so on. At this stage, the entire proposed CDiffE model can act as a complex environment for a higher agent-based model of WNV propagation including humans. In such an ABM, human agents can move through the CDiffE grid and may get infected. An extension of this chapter is studying the dynamics of the human component in such an ABM.

While, the next fundamental stage of this research is constructing and analyzing the above-mentioned ABM, many other areas are left open to improve upon. The results presented here may not be most optimum outcomes of the system. In this regards, a genetic algorithm with its superior ability to escape from local optima, due to its mutation operator, can be employed in the calibration process. The simulated annealing algorithm with its strengths in combinatorial problems could be also used in the calibration process to find the best combination of equation parameters. Furthermore, upon availability of quantitative data regarding the infected mosquito pools or birds, the infection-related parameters can be tuned. Currently these parameters, including biting rates and transmission parameters, are taken or estimated from other studies.

More recent publications by entomologists and ornithologists on bird viremia and their WNV-competence can always be adopted to further tune the estimates of corresponding parameters. One essential limitation with the proposed model is the implicit assumption of having the same virus transmission probabilities form different bird species to mosquitoes. A meaningful extension of current model is incorporating various transmission probabilities from birds to mosquitoes. Such an extension can be achieved by changing equation (3) as follows

$$M_s(t+1) = (1-\mu_m)\left[\prod_j (1-\beta_m^j)^{\frac{b^j B_i^j(t)}{H_t(t)+\Sigma_j B_t^j(t)}}\right] M_s(t) + (1-\mu_m)\,\gamma\, M_a(t)$$

where β^j_m is the virus transmission probability from bird species j to mosquitoes.

Improvement on initialization methods for the mosquito populations including the adult-stage and infected mosquito could be another possible direction for future work. Such methods may help change the model from a seasonal model to a year-around powerful simulation tool.

Lastly, the model does provide the capability to apply the impact of land cover/use on mosquito breeding rates. However, our collected data regarding the land cover parameter, L, may not have suitable values to describe the capacity of an environment for mosquito production. More practical discussions and remedy for this particular parameter is given in the Appendix.

ACKNOWLEDGMENTS

The authors thank Alex Reimer for help in collecting, parsing and compiling birds, weather and trap count dataset; the Manitoba Health Dept.,

Richard Baydack, Scott Graham-Derham, and Colleen Dudar for input on the trap data in Manitoba; Ryan Neighbour for consultation on designing difference equation and optimizing agent-based model structure; Ahmed Abdelrazec for consultation on designing difference equation; Christian Artuso for great input on collecting bird species traits and population estimates; Marm Kilpatrick for great input on estimating bird competence indices and other WNV-related parameters; Nick Komar for insightful comments on estimating bird WNV-related parameters and formulating mosquitos biting rates; Bernard Moulin for input on bird roosting locations, assumptions, and agent-based model structure; Bill Reisen for consultation and input on mosquito habitat preference and host seeking activities; Tasha Epp for input on prairie and bird roosting data in Canada; Phil Curry for helpful input on *Culex* species and regional coordinators in Manitoba; Sarah Bowden for input on land cover correlation with WNV; David Giffen and Agriculture and Agri-Food Canada for input on degree-day map.

AVAILABILITY OF DATA AND MATERIAL

The datasets supporting the conclusions of this chapter are included within the Nasrinpour et al.'s [24] and/or the Appendix.

REFERENCES

[1] Smithburn, K. C., T. P. Hughes, A. W. Burke, and J. H. Paul. "A Neurotropic Virus Isolated From the Blood of a Native of Uganda." *Amercian Journal of Tropical Medicine & Hygiene* s1-20, no. 4 (1940): 471–92.

[2] Nash, Denis, Farzad Mostashari, Annie Fine, James Miller, Daniel O'leary, Kristy Murray, Ada Huang et al. "The Outbreak of West Nile Virus Infection in the New York City Area in 1999." *New England Journal of Medicine* 344 (2001): 1807–14.

[3] Tachiiri, Kaoru, Brian Klinkenberg, Sunny Mak, and Jamil Kazmi. "Predicting Outbreaks: A Spatial Risk Assessment of West Nile Virus in British Columbia." *International Journal of Health Geography* 5 (2006): 21.

[4] Government of Manitoba. *Surveillance for West Nile virus in Manitoba. Manitoba Health, Seniors and Active Living.* Accessed April 15, 2015. http://www.gov.mb.ca/health/wnv/stats.html.

[5] Hayes, Edward B., Nicholas Komar, Roger S. Nasci, Susan P. Montgomery, Daniel R. O'Leary, and Grant L. Campbell. "Epidemiology and Transmission Dynamics of West Nile Virus Disease." *Emerging Infectious Diseases* 11 (2005): 1167–73. doi:10.3201/eid1108.050289a.

[6] Colpitts, Tonya M., Michael J. Conway, Ruth R. Montgomery, and Erol Fikrig. "West Nile Virus: Biology, Transmission, and Human Infection." *Clinical Microbioogy Review* 25 (2012): 635–48.

[7] Kramer, Laura D., Linda M. Styer, and Gregory D. Ebel. "A Global Perspective on the Epidemiology of West Nile Virus." *Annual REview of Entomology* 53 (2008): 61–81.

[8] Nasrinpour, Hamid Reza, Robert D. McLeod, and Marcia R. Friesen. "Agent Based Modelling and West Nile Virus: a Survey." *Journal of Medical and Biological Engineering* 39, no. 2 (2019): 178-183.

[9] Thomas, D. M., and B. Urena. "A Model Describing the Evolution of West Nile-like Encephalitis in New York City." *Mathematical and Computer Modeling* 34 (2001): 771–81.

[10] Wonham, Marjorie J., Tomas de-Camino-Beck, and Mark A. Lewis. "An Epidemiological Model for West Nile Virus: Invasion Analysis and Control Applications." *Proceedings of the Royal Society B: Biological Sciences* 271 (2004): 501–7.

[11] Bowman, C., A. B. Gumel, P. van den Driessche, J. Wu, and H. Zhu. "A Mathematical Model for Assessing Control Strategies Against West Nile Virus." *Bulletin of Mathematical Biology* 67 (2005): 1107–33. doi:10.1016/j.bulm.2005.01.002.

[12] Cruz-Pacheco, Gustavo, Lourdes Esteva, Juan Antonio Montaño-Hirose, and Cristobal Vargas. "Modelling the Dynamics of West Nile

Virus." *Bulletin of Mathematical Biology* 67 (2005): 1157–72. doi:10.1016/j.bulm.2004.11.008.
[13] Simpson, Jennifer E., Paul J. Hurtado, Jan Medlock, Goudarz Molaei, Theodore G. Andreadis, Alison P. Galvani, and Maria A. Diuk-Wasser. "Vector Host-feeding Preferences Drive Transmission of Multi-Host Pathogens: West Nile Virus as a Model System." *Proceedings of the Royal Society B: Biological Sciences* 279 (2012): 925–33.
[14] Chevalier, Véronique, Annelise Tran, and Benoit Durand. "Predictive Modeling of West Nile Virus Transmission Risk in the Mediterranean Basin: How Far From Landing?" *International Journal of Environmental Research and public Health* 11 (2013): 67–90.
[15] Nasrinpour, Hamid Reza, Marcia R. Friesen, and Robert D. McLeod. "An Agent-Based Model of Message Propagation in the Facebook Electronic Social Network." arXiv:161107454 [csSI]. 2016. http://arxiv.org/abs/1611.07454.
[16] Funk, Sebastian, Marcel Salathé, and Vincent AA Jansen. "Modelling the Influence of Human Behaviour on the Spread of Infectious Diseases: A Review." *Journal of the Royal Society Interface* 7 (2010).
[17] Salathé, Marcel, and James H. Jones. "Dynamics and Control of Diseases in Networks with Community Structure." *PLoS Computational Biology* 6:e1000736 (2010). doi:10.1371/journal.pcbi.1000736.
[18] Friesen, Marcia R. and Robert D. McLeod. "A Survey of Agent-Based Modeling of Hospital Environments." *IEEE Access* 2 (2014): 227–33. doi:10.1109/ACCESS.2014.2313957.
[19] Laskowski, Marek, Bryan C. P. Demianyk, Julia Witt, Shamir N. Mukhi, Marcia R. Friesen, and Robert D. McLeod. "Agent-Based Modeling of the Spread of Influenza-like Illness in an Emergency Department: A Simulation Study." *IEEE Transactions on Information Technology in Biomedicine* 15 (2011): 877–89. doi:10.1109/TITB.2011.2163414.
[20] Neighbour, Ryan, Luis Oppenheimer, Shamir N. Mukhi, Marcia R. Friesen, and Robert D. McLeod. "Agent Based Modeling of

"Crowdinforming" as a Means of Load Balancing at Emergency Departments." *Online Journal of Public Health Informatics* 2 (2010). doi:10.5210/ojphi.v2i3.3225.

[21] Silverman, Barry G., Nancy Hanrahan, Gnana Bharathy, Kim Gordon, and Dan Johnson. "A Systems Approach to Healthcare: Agent-based Modeling, Community Mental Health, and Population Well-being." *Artificial Intelligence in Medicine* 63 (2015): 61–71. doi:10.1016/j.artmed.2014.08.006.

[22] Li, Z., J. Hayse, I. Hlohowskyj, K. Smith, and R. Smith. "Agent-based Model for Simulation of West Nile Virus Transmission." *The Agent 2005 Conference on Generative Social Processes, Models, and Mechanisms* (2005): 459–72. http://mysite.science.uottawa.ca/rsmith43/AgentbasedmodelWNV.pdf.

[23] Bouden, Mondher, Bernard Moulin, and Pierre Gosselin. "The Geosimulation of West Nile Virus Propagation: A Multi-agent and Climate Sensitive Tool for Risk Management in Public Health." *International Journal of Health Geographics* 7 (2008): 35.

[24] Nasrinpour, Hamid R., Alex A. Reimer, Marcia R. Friesen, and Robert D. McLeod. "Data Preparation for West Nile Virus Agent-Based Modelling: Protocol for Processing Bird Population Estimates and Incorporating ArcMap in AnyLogic." *JMIR Research Protocols* 6:e138 (2017). doi:10.2196/resprot.6213.

[25] BAM Project Team. *BAM Effective Detection Radius. Boreal Avian Modelling Project* (2010). http://www.borealbirds.ca/index.php/bam_edr. Accessed 17 May 2016.

[26] Lewis, Mark A., Joanna Renclawowicz, P. van Den Driessche, and Marjorie Wonham. "A Comparison of Continuous and Discrete-time West Nile Virus Models." *Bulletin of Mathematical Biology* 68 (2006): 491–509.

[27] Abdelrazec, Ahmed, and Abba B. Gumel. "Mathematical Assessment of the Role of Temperature and Rainfall on Mosquito Population Dynamics." *Journal of Mathematical Biology* 42 (2016). doi:10.1007/s00285-016-1054-9.

[28] Government of Manitoba. *Land Use / Land Cover, Manitoba Land Initiative.* http://mli2.gov.mb.ca/landuse/index.html. Accessed September 29, 2015.

[29] Komar, Nicholas, Stanley Langevin, Steven Hinten, Nicole Nemeth, Eric Edwards, Danielle Hettler, Brent Davis, Richard Bowen, and Michel Bunning. "Experimental Infection of North American Birds with the New York 1999 Strain of West Nile Virus." *Emerging Infectious Diseases* 9 (2003): 311–22.

[30] Kilpatrick, A. Marm, Shannon L. LaDeau, and Peter P. Marra. "Ecology of West Nile Virus Transmission and its Impact on Birds in the Western Hemisphere." *The Auk* 124 (2007): 1121–36. doi:10.1642/0004-8038(2007)124[1121:EOWNVT]2.0.CO;2.

[31] Kilpatrick, A. Marm, Ryan J. Peters, Alan P. Dupuis II, Matthew J. Jones, Peter Daszak, Peter P. Marra, and Laura D. Kramer. "Predicted and Observed Mortality from Vector-borne Disease in Small Songbirds." *Biological Conservation* 165 (2013): 79–85. doi:10.1016/j.biocon.2013.05.015.

[32] Reisen, William K., and D. Caldwell Hahn. "Comparison of Immune Responses of Brown-headed Cowbird and Related Blackbirds to West Nile and other Mosquito-borne Encephalitis Viruses." *Journal of Wildlife Diseases* 43 (2007): 439–49. doi:10.7589/0090-3558-43.3.439.

[33] Reisen, W. K., Y. Fang, and V. M. Martinez. "Avian Host and Mosquito (Diptera: Culicidae) Vector Competence Determine the Efficiency of West Nile and St. Louis Encephalitis Virus Transmission." *Journal of Medical Entomology* 42 (2005): 367–75. http://www.ncbi.nlm.nih.gov/pubmed/15962789.

[34] Nemeth, Nicole, Daniel Gould, Richard Bowen, and Nicholas Komar. "Natural and Experimental West Nile Virus Infection in Five Raptor Species." *Journal of Wildlife Diseases* 42 (2006): 1–13. doi:10.7589/0090-3558-42.1.1.

[35] Fang, Ying, and William K. Reisen. "Previous Infection with West Nile or St. Louis Encephalitis Viruses Provides Cross Protection during Reinfection in House Finches." *American Journal of Tropical*

Medicine and *Hygiene* 75 (2006): 480–5. http://www.ncbi.nlm.nih.gov/pubmed/16968925.

[36] Reisen, William K., Ying Fang, and Vincent Martinez. "Is Nonviremic Transmission of West Nile Virus by Culex Mosquitoes (Diptera: Culicidae) Nonviremic?" *Journal of Medical Entomology* 44 (2007): 299–302. http://www.ncbi.nlm.nih.gov/pubmed/17427700.

[37] Komar, Nicholas, Nicholas A. Panella, Stanley A. Langevin, Aaron C. Brault, Manuel Amador, Eric Edwards, and Jennifer C. Owen. "Avian Hosts for West Nile Virus in St. Tammany Parish, Louisiana, 2002." *American Journal* of *Tropical Medicine* and *Hygiene* 73 (2005): 1031–7. http://www.ncbi.nlm.nih.gov/pubmed/16354808.

[38] Langevin, Stanley A., Aaron C. Brault, Nicholas A. Panella, Richard A. Bowen, and Nicholas Komar. "Variation in Virulence of West Nile Virus Strains for House Sparrows (Passer domesticus)." *American Journal* of *Tropical Medicine* and *Hygiene* 72 (2005): 99–102. http://www.ncbi.nlm.nih.gov/pubmed/15728874.

[39] Reisen, W. K., A. C. Brault, V. M. Martinez, Y. Fang, K. Simmons, S. Garcia, E. Omi-Olsen, and R. S. Lane. "Ability of Transstadially Infected Ixodes Pacificus (Acari: Ixodidae) to Transmit West Nile Virus to Song Sparrows or Western Fence Lizards." *Journal of Medical Entomology* 44 (2007): 320–7. http://www.ncbi.nlm.nih.gov/pubmed/17427704.

[40] Clark, Larry, Jeffrey Hall, Robert McLean, Michael Dunbar, Kaci Klenk, Richard Bowen, and Cynthia A. Smeraski. "Susceptibility of Greater Sage-Grouse to Experimental Infection with West Nile Virus." *Journal of Wildlife Diseases* 42 (2006): 14–22. doi:10.7589/0090-3558-42.1.14.

[41] Godsey, Marvin S., Kristen Burkhalter, Mark Delorey, and Harry M. Savage. "Seasonality and Time of Host-Seeking Activity of Culex Tarsalis and Floodwater Aedes in Northern Colorado, 2006-2007." *Journal of the American Mosquito Control Association* 26 (2010):148–59. doi:10.2987/09-5966.1.

[42] Reisen, W. K., H. D. Lothrop, and R. P. Meyer. "Time of Host-seeking by Culex tarsalis (Diptera:Culicidae) in California." *Journal of*

Medical Entomology 34 (1997): 430–7. http://www.ncbi.nlm.nih.gov/pubmed/9220677.

[43] Krebs, Bethany L., Tavis K. Anderson, Tony L. Goldberg, Gabriel L. Hamer, Uriel D. Kitron, Christina M. Newman, Marilyn O. Ruiz, Edward D. Walker, and Jeffrey D. Brawn. "Host Group Formation Decreases Exposure to Vector-borne Disease: A Field Experiment in a "Hotspot" of West Nile Virus transmission." *Proceedings of the Royal Society B: Biological Sciences* 281 (2014). http://rspb.royalsocietypublishing.org/content/281/1796/20141586.

[44] Janousek, William M., Peter P. Marra, and A. Marm Kilpatrick. "Avian Roosting Behavior Influences Vector-host Interactions for West Nile Virus Hosts." *Parasites and Vectors* 7 (2014): 399. doi:10.1186/1756-3305-7-399.

[45] Nasrinpour, Hamid, Amir Bavani, and Mohammad Teshnehlab. "Grouped Bees Algorithm: A Grouped Version of the Bees Algorithm." *Computers* 6 (2017). doi:10.3390/computers6010005.

[46] Laguna, Manuel. *Optimization of complex systems with OptQuest*. University of Colorado (1997). http://citeseerx.ist.psu.edu/viewdoc/summary?doi=10.1.1.120.6463.

[47] Pan, Leilei, Lixu Qin, Simon X. Yang, and Jiangping Shuai. "A Neural Network-Based Method for Risk Factor Analysis of West Nile Virus." *Risk Analysis* 28 (2008): 487–96. doi:10.1111/j.1539-6924.2008.01029.x.

[48] Denlinger, David L. and Peter A. Armbruster. "Mosquito Diapause." *Annual Review of Entomology* 59 (2014): 73–93. doi:10.1146/annurev-ento-011613-162023.

[49] Ruiz, Marilyn O., Luis F. Chaves, Gabriel L. Hamer, Ting Sun, William M. Brown, Edward D. Walker, Linn Haramis, Tony L. Goldberg, and Uriel D. Kitron. "Local Impact of Temperature and Precipitation on West Nile Virus Infection in Culex Species Mosquitoes in Northeast Illinois, USA." *Parasites and Vectors* 3 (2010): 19. doi:10.1186/1756-3305-3-19.

[50] Paull, Sara H., Daniel E. Horton, Moetasim Ashfaq, Deeksha Rastogi, Laura D. Kramer, Noah S. Diffenbaugh, and A. Marm Kilpatrick.

"Drought and Immunity Determine the Intensity of West Nile Virus Epidemics and Climate Change Impacts." *Proceedings of the Royal Society B: Biological Sciences* 284 (2017): 20162078. doi:10.1098/rspb.2016.2078.

[51] Cooke, William H., Katarzyna Grala, and Robert C. Wallis. "Avian GIS Models Signal Human Risk for West Nile Virus in Mississippi." *International Journal of Health Geographics* 5 (2006): 36.

[52] Dieng, Hamady, GM Saifur Rahman, A. Abu Hassan, MR Che Salmah, Tomomitsu Satho, Fumio Miake, Michael Boots, and AbuBakar Sazaly. "The Effects of Simulated Rainfall on Immature Population Dynamics of Aedes albopictus and Female Oviposition." *International Journal of Biometereology* 56 (2012): 113–20.

[53] Epstein, Paul R., and Caroline Defilippo. "West Nile Virus and Drought." *Global Change and Human Health* 2, no. 2 (2001): 105–7. http://dx.doi.org/10.1023/A:1015089901425.

[54] Shaman, Jeffrey, Jonathan F. Day, and Marc Stieglitz. "Drought-induced Amplification and Epidemic Transmission of West Nile Virus in Southern Florida." *Journal of Medical Entomology* 42 (2005): 134–41.

[55] American Mosquito Control Association. *Mosquito Life Cycle*. http://www.mosquito.org/life-cycle. Accessed April 15, 2015. http://www.webcitation.org/6iJntDZde.

[56] Cornel, Anton J., Peter G. Jupp, and Nigel K. Blackburn. "Environmental Temperature on the Vector Competence of Culex univittatus (Diptera: Culicidae) for West Nile Virus." *Journal of Medical Entomology* 30 (1993): 449–56. http://www.ncbi.nlm.nih.gov/pubmed/8459423.

[57] Dohm, David J., Monica L. O'Guinn, and Michael J. Turell. "Effect of Environmental Temperature on the Ability of Culex pipiens (Diptera: Culicidae) to Transmit West Nile Virus." *Journal of Medical Entomology* 39 (2002): 221–5. http://www.ncbi.nlm.nih.gov/pubmed/11931261.

[58] Reisen, William K., Daniel Cayan, Mary Tyree, Christopher M. Barker, Bruce Eldridge, and Michael Dettinger. "Impact of Climate

Variation on Mosquito Abundance in California." *Journal of Vector Ecology* 33 (2008): 89–98.

[59] Reisen, William K., Ying Fang, and Vincent M. Martinez. "Effects of Temperature on the Transmission of West Nile Virus by Culex tarsalis (Diptera: Culicidae). *Journal of Medical Entomology* 43 (2006): 309–17. doi:10.1603/0022-2585(2006)043[0309:eotott]2.0.co;2.

[60] Dodson, Brittany L., Laura D. Kramer, and Jason L. Rasgon. "Effects of Larval Rearing Temperature on Immature Development and West Nile Virus Vector Competence of Culex tarsalis." *Parasites and Vectors* 5 (2012): 199. doi:10.1186/1756-3305-5-199.

[61] Chen, Chen-Chih, Tasha Epp, Emily Jenkins, Cheryl Waldner, Philip Curry, and Catherine Soos. "Modeling Monthly Variation of Culex tarsalis (Diptera: Culicidae) Abundance and West Nile Virus Infection Rate in the Canadian Prairies." *International Journal of Environmental Research and Public Health* 10 (2013): 3033–51.

[62] Manore, Carrie A., Kyle S. Hickmann, James M. Hyman, Ivo M. Foppa, Justin K. Davis, Dawn M. Wesson, and Christopher N. Mores. "A Network-patch Methodology for Adapting Agent-based Models for Directly Transmitted Disease to Mosquito-borne Disease." *Journal of Biological Dynamics* 9 (2015): 52–72. doi:10.1080/17513758.2015.1005698.

APPENDIX

Introduction

This Appendix provides additional detail on the work found in the main chapter. Specifically, the Appendix provides additional review of the literature on the problem at hand, and provides additional details, characterization, and explanation of the mathematical parameters applied in this work. The Appendix supports the validity of the work in the main chapter, and may be of most interest to those who may be interested in replicating the work.

In North America, at least 59 different species of mosquitoes [1, 2] and over 225 species of birds [3, 4] have been found infected with WNV. However, not all of the mosquito species act as bridge vectors by feeding on both birds and mammals (including humans). There are several studies with data on different mosquito species and bridge vectors [5–7]. Only some mosquito genera have been reported in each area of the world, and their population count heavily depends on weather conditions and landscape features [8].

Avian hosts are believed to be responsible for large-scale spread of WNV mainly due to their food seeking activities and somewhat migration [9, 10]. Traits and behaviour (e.g., roosting) of each species of birds play an important role in prevalence of WNV [11–13]. Among birds, some species such as *corvidae*, commonly referred to as the crow family, are known to be competent hosts. The crows become severely ill after the infection and often die, whereas many others do not become ill and develop WNV antibodies to resist against infection [14]. Host competence is typically determined by the duration and magnitude of viremia. The contribution of different bird species to WNV transmission to mosquitoes is determined by the combination of competence, abundance, and mosquito feeding patterns. Several studies have quantitatively determined which host species are more important in different parts of North America [15, 16]. Many other studies offers insights on mosquito feeding patterns and the role of different bird species (and their community structure) in WNV amplification [17–20].

Mosquito species differ in their preferred breeding habitats, biting behaviour, flight range, life-cycle period, host preference, etc. It is believed that differences in mosquito habitat preferences may be the reason why both extreme (wet and dry) weather conditions result in outbreaks [21]. A more recent study on weather drivers of WNV across North America can be found in the work of Paull et al. [22]. The *Culex* (*Cx.*) *pipiens* is the main competent WNV vector in the eastern United States and Canada including southern Ontario and Quebec [2, 4] and is one of the most important vectors capable of amplifying WNV in the bird population [23]. These primarily bird biting mosquitoes are mostly found in urban areas and have habitat preferences of water with high organic content [21, 24, 25]. *Cx. quinquefasciatus* is also important in the southeastern part of the United States [26]. *Cx. restuans* mosquito is another competent primarily bird biting vector for WNV. Its biting activity is mainly at night, and has a similar breeding habitat as *Cx. pipiens*. The *Cx. tarsalis* mosquitoes are extremely efficient in preserving and intensifying WNV and considered to be the main vector in the Prairie provinces of Alberta, Manitoba and Saskatchewan [4, 27–29]. This species, similar to other *Cx.* species, can transmit WNV to its offspring [30]. It feeds multiple times on mostly birds and sometimes mammals [4, 31]. The larvae of this principal bridge vector in Manitoba can tolerate a wide range of water conditions [32]. The species can be found in almost any fresh water source except tree holes, including temporary water bodies (e.g., bird baths and used tires), alkaline lakes, and salty wetlands [4, 32, 33]. Larval habitat can be shared with other species such as *Cx. pipiens* and several species of *Aedes* and *Anopheles* [32]. A female can produce eggs multiple times during a season [4, 33], although up to 95% of larvae can be lost by predation [32]. The life cycle duration depends on temperature, lasting approximately 14 days at 21° C and only 10 days at 26°C [34]. They are reported to be persistent biters at dusk and even during the day [4, 35, 36]. Their foraging flight is typically less than one kilometer, but it can be extended well beyond six kilometers up to 27 km [23, 32]. The combination of traits that characterizes *Cx. tarsalis* are essential knowledge when developing transmission models.

Methods

Weather and Landscape Impacts

The daily update equations for reproduction per time-unit, r, hourly maturation probability, γ, and hourly probability of natural death of aquatic and adult mosquitoes, μ_a and μ_m, in the core Difference Equation (DiffE) are as follows.

$$r = r(T, R, L) = \left[\alpha_b e^{-a_b (T-T_b)^2}\right] \left[\frac{(1+s_b)\, e^{-r_b(R-R_b)^2}}{e^{-r_b(R-R_b)^2} + s_b}\right] [1 + w_L L]$$

$$\gamma = \gamma(T, R) = \left[\alpha_d e^{-a_d (T-T_d)^2}\right] \left[\frac{(1+s_d)\, e^{-r_d(R-R_d)^2}}{e^{-r_d(R-R_d)^2} + s_d}\right]$$

$$\mu_a = \mu_a(T, R) = [c_a(T - T_a)^2 + d_a]\left[1 + \frac{e_a R}{1+R}\right]$$

$$\mu_m = \mu_m(T) = [c_m(T - T_m)^2 + d_m]$$

where T and R are daily temperature and rainfall at time-step t. Temperature is truncated to be always positive. L is a special linear combination of land cover correlations of a mosquito site, which will be explained shortly; and the parameter w_L basically indicates the importance of land cover of a mosquito site. The rest of parameters in this set of functions controls how the temperature and rainfall-dependent functions react to the variations of weather conditions. A discussion of these parameters can be found in [37]. For the scope of this paper, it is only important to tune these parameters according to the weather and mosquito surveillance data in Southern Manitoba.

In addition to the functions above, the mosquitoes biting rate (i.e., number per unit of time) is also a function of temperature and host preference. The host preference is added to the model by multiplying a coefficient between zero and one to the mosquitoes biting rate. The effect of temperature on (hourly) biting rate is controlled through the following equation from [38].

$$b = b(T) = \frac{1}{24} \lfloor -0.00014\, T^2 + 0.027\, T - 0.322 \rfloor^+$$

where

$$\lfloor f(x) \rfloor^+ = \begin{cases} f(x) & ; if\ f(x) > 0 \\ 0 & ; otherwise \end{cases}$$

According to the Manitoba Land Initiative [39], there are 18 known classes and one unknown class of land cover identified in our land cover/use dataset. On the other hand, Bowden et al. [40] report Pearson correlations between 14 types of land cover and West Nile Virus disease incidence in humans in the United States. The detailed description of their land cover types can be found in [41]. The Pearson correlation values and mapping from their types of land cover to our classes of land cover can be found in Table 1. These correlation values combined with the proportional areas of each type of land cover in our mosquito sites define the parameter L as follows:

$$L = \sum_i l_i \times p_i$$

where l_i is the proportional area of different land cover classes, and p_i is the Pearson correlation for each class of land cover. For example, the value of L for the mosquito site/cell in Figure 1 is as follows.

$$\begin{aligned}L_{Fig.1} &= 0.2\, p_{Residential} + 0.33\, p_{AgriculturalField} + 0.15\, p_{Rocks} + 0.32\, p_{WaterBody} \\ &= 20\% \times (-0.19) + 33\% \times 0.3 + 15\% \times (-0.05) + 32\% \times 0 = 0.0535\end{aligned}$$

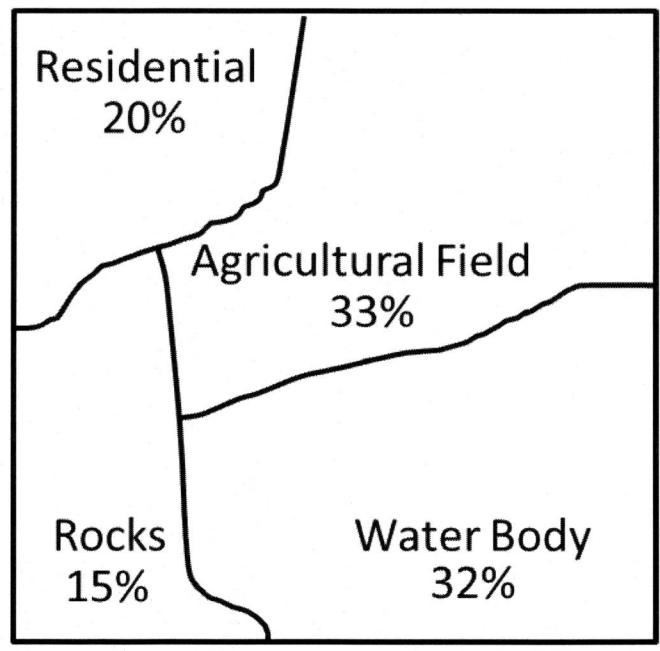

Figure A1. An example of land use/cover classes in a mosquito cell/site.

Multiple Bird Species and Rates

Before describing how the current implementation of the proposed CDiffE model differentiates between various bird species, a few facts and assumptions are reviewed:

1. For most species, susceptibility to infection is 100% [42], that is, we can assume that the transmission probability from an infected mosquito to a bird is 100%. To be clear, this virus transmission makes a bird infected, but not all the infected birds become infectious.
2. There is no infected bird compartment in our proposed difference equation model, but only the infectious bird state. This means a bird is marked as infectious only if the infected bird has the competency to transmit the virus to another mosquito vector. Otherwise, the infected bird remains a susceptible bird in the model.
3. There are studies on the reservoir competence index value of an infected bird, which describes the relative proportion of vector mosquitoes that become infectious after feeding on such a bird [42, 43]. These data could help directly estimate the probability of transmission from bird to mosquito, given the contact rate.
4. Our difference equation model as currently formulated, does not differentiate (i.e., per bird species) virus transmission probabilities from bird to mosquito. That is β_m cannot be a vector or an array. Removing this assumption is discussed in the main paper.
5. For the estimation of mosquito contact rate with each bird species, host-seeking mosquitoes' **abundance data** and dynamic WNV data are necessary. Unfortunately, we did not have access to these data from Manitoba. Additionally, host preference of *Culex tarsalis* mosquitoes depends on the species available in a region [44], i.e., *Cx. tarsalis* mosquitoes have opportunistic host-seeking habits [45, 46].

Considering the facts 1 – 4, the virus transmission probability from bird to mosquito (i.e., β_m) is the same for all bird species, and the virus transmission probability from mosquito to bird (i.e., β_b) is adjusted based on the reservoir competence index for each bird species. That is:

$$\begin{cases} \forall_j \ \beta_m^j = \beta_m \\ \beta_b^j = c^j \beta_b \end{cases}$$

where c^j is the host competence index for the bird species j. A host competence index is a metric to indicate relative number of mosquitoes which become infectious as a result of biting the infected host [42, 43].

Given the fact 5, and the tendency to lower the computational complexity of the model, in our implementation, the biting rate (i.e., the number of bites made per mosquito per time step) is the same among different bird species; and humans' biting rate is a proportion of birds' biting rate. That is:

$$\begin{cases} \forall_j \ b^j = b \\ b_h = \frac{1}{\lambda} b \end{cases}$$

where λ is the ratio of mosquito biting activities on birds to biting activities on humans.

The next two parameters to calculate for birds species are recovery, ζ_b, and death due to infection, δ, probabilities per unit of time. The procedure to estimate these two probabilities and associated rates are explained in another section.

Bird Species' Competence Index

In the DiffE model, host competence indices are used as weights to adjust the virus transmission probability (i.e., β_b) for each species. Basically, if the host viremia is less than an infectious threshold in a day, its infectiousness is set at zero for the day. If not, the infectiousness is calculated. The average daily infectiousness of birds of the same species is then summed over the viremic period to produce the species index [43]. The infectiousness threshold used in these studies is for *Cx. pipiens* mosquitoes, and in general *Cx. tarsalis* mosquitoes are competent at a lower viremia level. However, the threshold is not as important as the fraction of infectious mosquitoes used in the calculation of species index [43]. Besides, these competence indices are normalized and used as relative weights. So the resulting effect on the difference equation model will be almost the same. For bird species that had not been tested, the average values from other species of the same family or order were used. Strictly speaking, for most of missing species, the order average was used except for a few Passeriformes where some data for the family was available. Normalized host competence indices for some of the birds' species can be found in Table 2.

Bird Species' Recovery and Death Rates and Probabilities

To begin with, assume the experimental studies are available for a species. In this case, for each species the following information could be obtained from the literature [42, 43]; the fraction of birds who died, (p_d), the fraction of birds who recovered, (p_r), the average number of days to death, (n_d), and the average number of days to recover from being infectious, (n_r). In other words, from a statistical perspective, the average probability of death is p_d for a period of n_d days, and the probability of recovery in an interval of n_r days is p_r on average.

It is important to recall that the difference equation model is formed in such a way that the events of death due to infection and recovery from infection are two independent events (see equation (6) from the main paper). This means infectious birds remain infectious if they do not die and at the same time do not recover. Therefore, in estimating each of these two hourly probabilities the impact of the other is disregarded. As such, it is reasonable to fit a Poisson model with rate parameter θ to the problem in order to determine the probability of number of death events (or recovery events) that occurred per unit of time. Let k_h be the number of events in an interval of h hours (or time-steps). Thus, the probability of n events occurring in h hours is given by the probability mass function (PMF) of a Poisson distribution as follows.

$$P(k_h = n) = Poisson(k_h; \theta h) = \frac{(\theta h)^{k_h} e^{-\theta h}}{k_h!} \qquad (A.1)$$

where θ is the hourly rate (i.e., expected number of events per time-step), and (θh) is the average number of events in h hours. Consequently, the probability of observing at least one event (e.g., death or recovery) per unit of time (i.e., $h = 1$) is given by

$$P(k_1 > 0) = 1 - P(k_1 = 0) = 1 - e^{-\theta} \qquad (A.2)$$

Now the information regarding each species from the literature can be applied to solve the equation (A.1) for θ, and the hourly probability is then given by equation (A.2). That is, if θ_d represents the hourly rate of dying due to infection, the probability of *not* dying due to infection in n_d days (i.e., $24n_d$ hours) is

$$P(k_{24n_d} = 0) = 1 - p_d = e^{-\theta_d(24n_d)}$$

where $0 \leq p_d < 1$ and $n_d > 0$ can be taken from the literature in [42]. This yields

$$\theta_d = -\frac{\ln(1-p_d)}{24n_d} \qquad (A.3)$$

As such, the hourly probability of dying due to infection, δ, and leaving the infectious state can be derived from the corresponding rate as

$$\delta = 1 - e^{-\theta_d} \qquad (A.4)$$

Similarly, if θ_r represents the hourly rate of recovery from infection, this rate will be calculated as

$$\theta_r = -\frac{\ln(1-p_r)}{24n_r} \qquad (A.5)$$

where $0 \leq p_r < 1$ and $n_r > 0$ can be taken from the literature in [42, 43]; and consequently, the hourly probability of recovery, ζ_b, and leaving the infectious state is derived from the corresponding rate as follows

$$\zeta_b = 1 - e^{-\theta_r} \tag{A.6}$$

For the corner case where $p_d = 1$ (and $p_r = 0$), i.e., all birds die due to infection (and no one recovers), the hourly recovery probability, ζ_b, is simply set to zero, but the hourly death probability, δ, is *not* set to one, thus avoiding changing the infectious birds' state in only one time-step as desired. Therefore, in this case, instead of using the equation (A.3), the hourly *rate* of dying due to infection, θ_d, in equation (A.4) is deliberately set to $1/24n_d$. That is

$$\delta = 1 - e^{-\frac{1}{24n_d}} \quad ; \quad \zeta_b = 0 \tag{A.7}$$

Similarly, for the corner case where $p_r = 1$ (and $p_d = 0$), i.e., when all birds recover from infectiousness (and no one dies), the hourly death probability, δ, is simply set to zero, but the hourly recovery probability, ζ_b, is not set to one. Herein, the recovery probability, ζ_b, is given by equation (A.6) where the recovery *rate* of θ_r takes the value of $1/24n_r$ instead of taking its value from the equation (A.5). That is

$$\zeta_b = 1 - e^{-\frac{1}{24n_r}} \quad ; \quad \delta = 0 \tag{A.8}$$

In summary, where the experimental studies are available for a species, death and recovery rates are estimated, and the corresponding probabilities are then calculated according to equations (A.1) - (A.6). Herein, the parameter n_r for species is set to the number of days that the species maintain a high level of viremia in their bloodstream to be infectious for mosquitoes. These values are taken from the data used in [43]. The other three parameters of p_d, p_r, and n_d are taken directly from [42] for a limited number of species. These values for a number of bird's species can be found in Table.

Where the experimental data are missing for a species, estimation of death and recovery rates for each species were made based on the following rules of thumbs and assumptions.

1. For bird species with no reported experimental studies, the average values from other species of the same family or order were used when there were some data available regarding at least one species in these orders/families.
2. Orders and families reported as incompetent in [47] were given a zero death rate, and one recovery rate; unless there was explicitly some data reported regarding at least one species in these orders/families. This assumption means incompetent birds do not die due to infection and will recover from infectiousness in one time-step.
3. When "no signs of clinical illness" were explicitly reported as in [42] for a certain order, a zero death rate was given to all their species; unless there were explicitly some data reported regarding at least one species in this order. This assumption means if birds of a certain order do not show any symptoms of the disease, they will not die due to infection.
4. In all other cases where there was no general information available regarding a certain order, the recovery rate of a species was set to the average recovery rate of all birds with known data. The death rate of species of these orders was assumed to be zero. This means birds of high WNV mortality such as passerines (and especially corvids) are assumed to be known. Therefore, birds with no experimental studies must have a negligible (or even zero) death rate. Even though these species may have been found dead while their bloodstream had an infection, yet one cannot confirm whether the death was a direct result of infection without proper experimental studies.

Hourly rates and probabilities of recovery from infectiousness and death due to infection for a number of birds' species can be found in Table 2.

Mosquito Nocturnal Activities

An average hourly biting probability should at least be split into high and low biting activity values for nights and days, respectively. Assuming the parameter $\bar{b}$ indicates the average hourly probability of biting for a certain species (or humans), the following equations derives the mosquito biting probabilities for nights and days based on daylight hours, D, in a given day and ratio of biting activities between nights and days, ω, such that the average hourly value holds true for a 24-hour day.

$$\begin{cases} \dfrac{b_{night}}{b_{day}} = \omega > 1 \\ \sum b_{night} + b_{day} = 24\bar{b} \end{cases} \Rightarrow Db_{day} + (24 - D)\omega b_{day} = 24\bar{b}$$

$$\Rightarrow \begin{cases} b_{day} = \dfrac{24}{(24 - D)\omega + D}\bar{b} \\ b_{night} = \omega b_{day} \end{cases}$$

where b_{day} and b_{night} are mosquito biting probabilities during days and nights, respectively. This means these two parameters would replace the parameter b in the equations (4) and (8) (and the parameter b_h in the equation (14)) from the main paper, based on the current hour of the day.

Table A1. Birds' species estimated parameters

Common name	c*	pd*	pr*	nd*	nr*	24θd*	δ*	24θr*	ζb*
Blue Jay	0.7565	75%	25%	4.7	4	0.295	0.01221	0.072	0.00299
American Crow	0.5931	100%	0%	5.1	N/A	0.196	0.00814	0	0
Common Grackle	0.4460	33%	67%	4.5	4	0.089	0.00370	0.277	0.01148
House Finch	0.4057	100%	0%	7	N/A	0.143	0.00593	0	0
House Sparrow	0.3917	50%	50%	4.7	5	0.147	0.00613	0.139	0.00576
Black-billed Magpie	0.3563	100%	0%	6	N/A	0.167	0.00692	0	0
American Robin	0.3287	-	-	-	3	0.112	0.00466	0.333	0.01379
Song Sparrow	0.3084	-	-	-	5	0.112	0.00466	0.200	0.00830
American Kestrel	0.2477	-	-	-	3	0	0	0.333	0.01379
Brewer's Blackbird	0.2177	-	-	-	4	0.044	0.00185	0.250	0.01036
Great Horned Owl	0.2133	-	-	-	4	0	0	0.250	0.01036
Red-tailed Hawk	0.1623	-	-	-	5	0	0	0.200	0.00830
Red-winged Blackbird	0.1349	-	-	-	3	0.044	0.00185	0.333	0.01379
Northern Mockingbird	0.0934	-	-	-	2	0.112	0.00466	0.500	0.02062
European Starling	0.0541	-	-	-	4	0.112	0.00466	0.250	0.01036
Northern Flicker	0.0452	-	-	-	2	0	0	0.500	0.02062
Swainson's Thrush	0.0376	-	-	-	1	0.112	0.00466	1	0.04081
Mourning Dove	0.0285	-	-	-	3	0	0	0.333	0.01379
Gray Catbird	0.0248	-	-	-	1	0.112	0.00466	1	0.04081
Rock Pigeon	0.0013	-	-	-	1	0	0	1	0.04081
Brown-headed Cowbird	0	-	-	-	1	0	0	1	0.04081
Ring-necked Pheasant	0	-	-	-	1	0	0	1	0.04081

* c: relative competence index; p_d: percent of birds who died due to infection;; p_r: percent of birds who recovered; n_d: mean number of days till death due to infection occurred; n_r: number of infectiosness days; $24\theta_d$: daily death rate; δ: hourly death probability; $24\theta_r$: daily recovery rate; ζ_b: hourly recovery probability.

Parameter Calibration and Model Validation

The obtained trap data in Manitoba [29] does not provide sufficient information regarding the number of infected mosquitoes for validation and tuning purposes, as the data only indicate if there is at least one infected mosquito in a given week in a community, and they do not provide any information about the number of infected pools. The data from 2004 to 2013 are used as training data for calibration and tuning purposes, and the data from 2014 is then used for validation as the test data. Alternatively, we could have performed a k-fold cross-validation on the limited available dataset by partitioning the data into different training and test years and averaging the results over all the rounds. This is often carried out in statistical prediction models, particularly when few data are available, and it would have been especially crucial if the intent was to report an accuracy report for a finalized software package for WNV prediction in Manitoba for all years. However, the calibration process was very time-consuming in this work. As well, the goal here was to achieve acceptable behaviour to proceed with the CDiffE or a higher ABM to study various scenarios. After performing the calibration procedure, for further simulations, either the test year or the average of all years was used.

There are two general choices for correlation calculations: Pearson and Spearman rank order. The Pearson correlation compares the absolute numbers. It is more sensitive to outliers, such as wrong trap data in this application, yet it uses most of the information available from the data. It is notable that other than many missing data, it was confirmed that some traps may had failed for various reasons for any given week. This information was not available in the obtained data though. Alternatively, Spearman rank order correlation does not need such accurate data, as it only considers the ranks (orders) of numbers. For example, as long as the model's output for week two is higher than week one and less than week three, and this is also the case in the trap data, the correlation is 100%. The Spearman rank correlation is only good to achieve the relative trend, and not the amplitude of changes. Therefore, the data over different communities for every single week were summed up and treated as the total count for each week. This figure is compared against the total density of mosquitoes in those communities in the model for each week to be used in the sensitive Pearson correlation; whereas the Spearman rank correlation was applied to compare every single pair of weeks and communities. A linear combination of both metrics with equal weights was chosen as the first fitness function. The second fitness function was the ratio between the total number of CDC trapped mosquitoes in a year, and the total mosquitoes generated in the simulation year. As such, the calibration algorithm had two key objectives: (1) maximizing the correlation, (2) minimizing the population difference. The weights of each of these two fitness functions for the correlation-oriented, population-oriented, and balanced-approach solutions are seven to three, three to seven, five to five, respectively.

The optimization process produced some solutions with excellent performance in some years, but very poor matching trends in other years. Therefore, a minor penalty was applied to the solutions where the correlation was negative in a year. This penalty was imposed to achieve a general solution for producing a fair result in all years from 2004 to 2013.

Results and Discussion

Calibration Results

For the scope of this paper, the human component is not yet added to the simulation implementations. This assumes H_t is zero in its all corresponding equations. The values of equation parameters for each of the three solutions are given in Table A2. The generally suggested values for daily rate of these parameters for an equivalent DE model is given in Table [37].

All the simulation runs were given an initial (small) number of 2000 × $(1 + w_L L)$ mosquitoes in each mosquito site in the CDC week no. 21 (i.e., approximately the last week of April). It is notable that the parameter α_b and w_L are the same in all solutions as the model is highly sensitive to changes on these two parameters (see [37] for a discussion on the sensitivity of model to the reproduction rate). Accounting for the impact of w_L, an α_b value of 12 is associated to a maximum of 288 eggs, laid by each adult female mosquito during a day which is in agreement with biological studies [48]. The second parameter of w_L defines the impact of landscape features on mosquito habitat. While it may have been expected to have a high value of close to one for w_L, its value was set at 0.1 by the optimizer. The reason can be explained via Figure where the parameter L (i.e., land use correlation with the number of WNV human cases) for Southern Manitoba is depicted.

Table A2. Numerical values of equation parameters for each of the three solutions of calibration process

	Correlation-oriented	Population-oriented	Balanced-approach
αb	12	12	12
ab	1E-5	1E-06	3.866E-6
Tb	22	25	24
sb	2	1.799	1.819
rb	0.006	0.008	0.009
rd	0.004	0.006	0.006
Td	23	26	25
Rb	20	20	17
ad	0.04	0.04	0.029
αd	1E-5	6.36E-05	1.671E-5
sd	2.245	3.655	3.774
Rd	22	18	17
ca	1E-10	1E-10	1.019E-10
da	1.36E-4	6.64E-05	1.688E-4
Ta	27	28	25
ea	0.001	0.0001	0.001
cm	1.474E-4	3.79E-05	4.587E-5
Tm	25	28	28
dm	2.725E-4	0.001	9.919E-4
wL	0.1	0.1	0.1

As shown in Figure A2, approximately the half of southern Manitoba (i.e., the area of interest of this study) has a negative correlation with WNV human cases in comparison to the whole North America. As such, high values of w_L could have significantly reduced the total number of mosquitoes generated in many grid cells, which is *not* desired and is penalized in the fitness function of the optimization process. So, a low positive value of 0.1 was selected by the optimizer as w_L to avoid underproduction of mosquitoes and to achieve a high Pearson correlation at the same time. However, if in a specific application the population census is not as important as having a higher Pearson correlation, the value of w_L could be carefully increased and fixed. Once the value of w_L is updated, an optimizing search for tuning other parameters is recommended though. A report on the variations of w_L is given in another section.

Table A3. Suggested values of the corresponding daily rates for some of the equation parameters from various sources as reported in [37]. Some values are derived based on the reported values in [37]

Parameter	Value	Parameter	Value	Parameter	Value
αb	300/day	Td	22 °C	ca	2.5E-9/day
ab	0.015/day	Rb	10 mm	da	0.015/day
Tb	22°C	ad	0.011 /day	Ta	20°C
sb	1.2/day	αd	0.0875/day	ea	1.1/day
rb	0.05/day	sd	1.5/day	cm	0.0005/day
rd	0.05/day	Rd	15 mm	Tm	28°C
dm	0.04/day	wL	N/A		

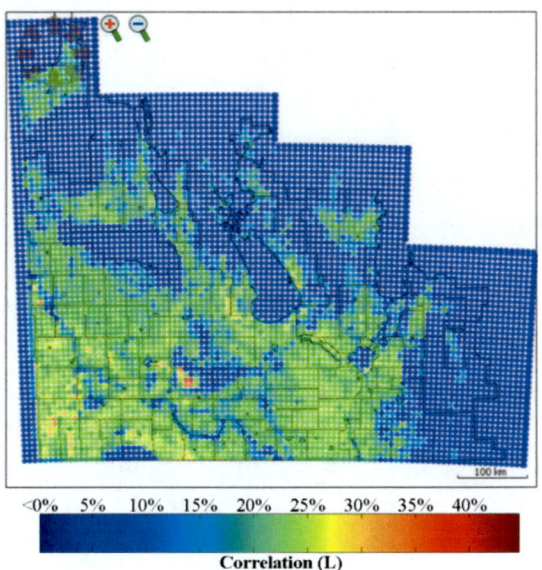

Figure A2. Weighted average land cover correlation with the number of WNV human cases (i.e., the parameter L) where the dark blue color denotes a non-positive correlation.

Generally, vegetation type and water bodies are the two main elements that need to be described by landscape variables or indexes. An alternative for land cover impacts in WNV modelling is to directly calculate mosquito-related indexes for the land. As an example, normalized difference vegetation index (NDV), which assess the land cover from a vegetation perspective with a numerical value between -1 and 1, has been identified and used as a risk factor for mosquito abundance models [21, 49, 50]. Other landscape parameters used in the WNV literature to describe mosquito habitat include stream density, slope percent, soil type, and distance to the nearest wetlands/bogs [10, 21, 49].

Model Validation

Supplementary to what presented in the main paper, Figure here shows degree day accumulation base 14.3°C [29, 51] for a simulation performed for 2014. The degree day function used in Figure is derived from [52].

Cumulative degree days map [51] are shown in Figure as the Manitoba government as well as many modellers explicitly employ degree days as an indicator of WNV activities. The reason is that the development of mosquitoes and the virus both need warm weather over a period of time. Degree-days index for a given day shows the number of degrees Celsius the mean temperature of the day is below or above a pre-defined base threshold. For *Cx. tarsalis* mosquitoes, the base number is estimated to be 14.3°C, and the activation of virus (extrinsic incubation period) requires 109 Degree-Days (DD) [53]. Reference [54] gives an example of degree days WNV models. Although degree days were not explicitly used in the proposed cellular model, the model output considers it to some extent. This confirms the importance of temperature on the mosquito life-cycle and WNV activities. The impact of temperature is explicitly assessed and reported in the main paper.

Sensitivity Report

Changes of the average of the three evaluation metrics for the balanced-approach solution in response to variations of w_L is plotted in Figure for all the years from 2004 to 2014. As shown in Figure , expectedly, the average Pearson correlation gradually rises as the value of w_L goes up to a maximum threshold of approximately 1.3, and then a marginal decreasing trend begins. For the low or even negative values of w_L, the Spearman rank-order correlation remains almost constant at around 50% followed by a sharp decrease beginning at a positive value of 0.2 for w_L; whereas the population scale has a steady declining trend as the value of w_L increases.

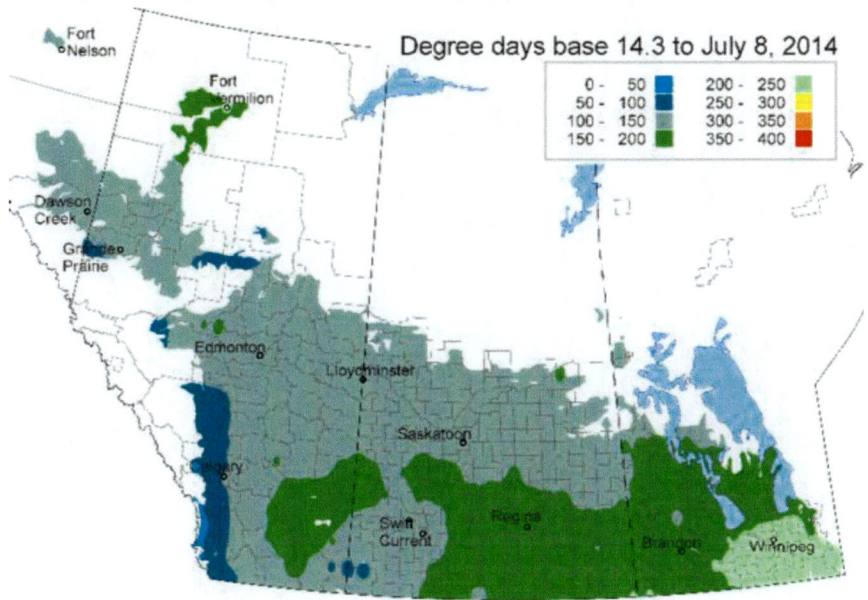

Week 27 in 2014

Figure 3. (Continued).

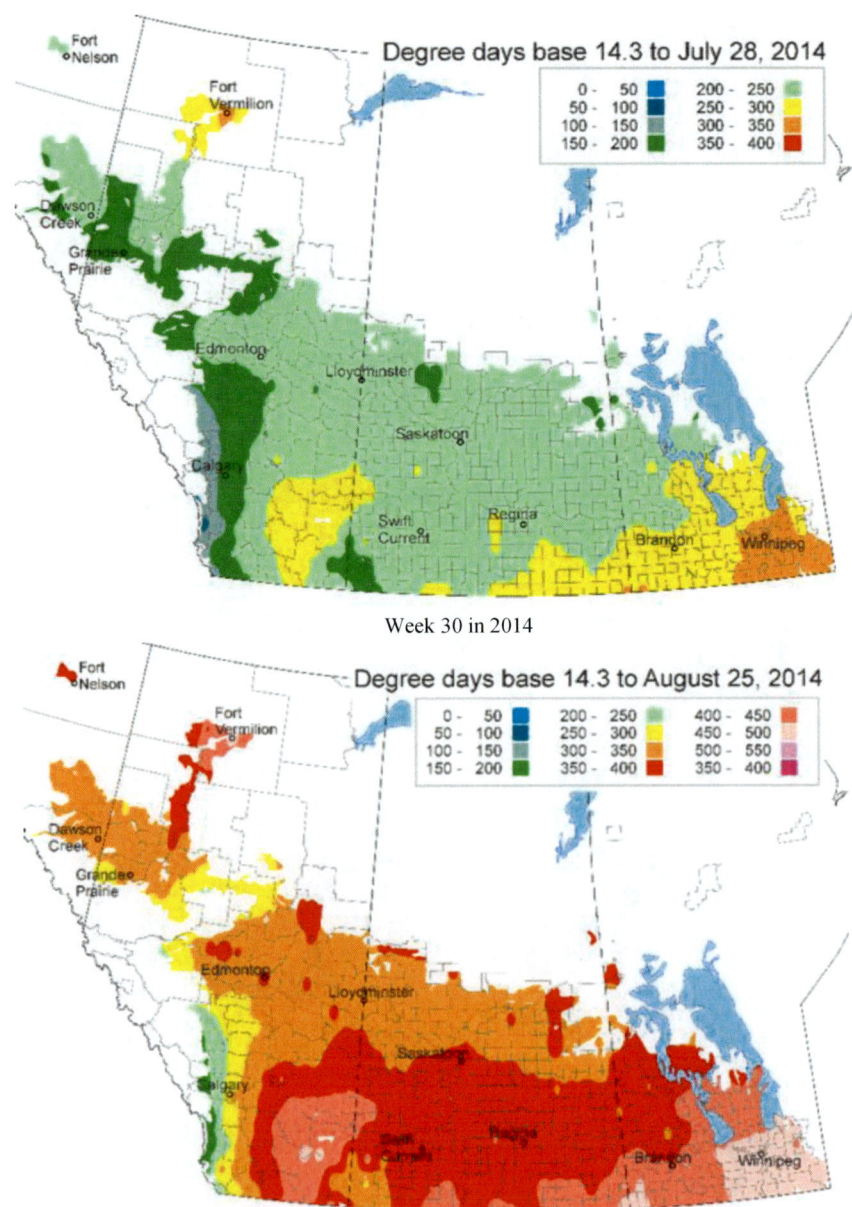

Week 30 in 2014

Source: Agriculture and Agri-Food Canada [51].

Figure 3. The map of cumulative degree-days.

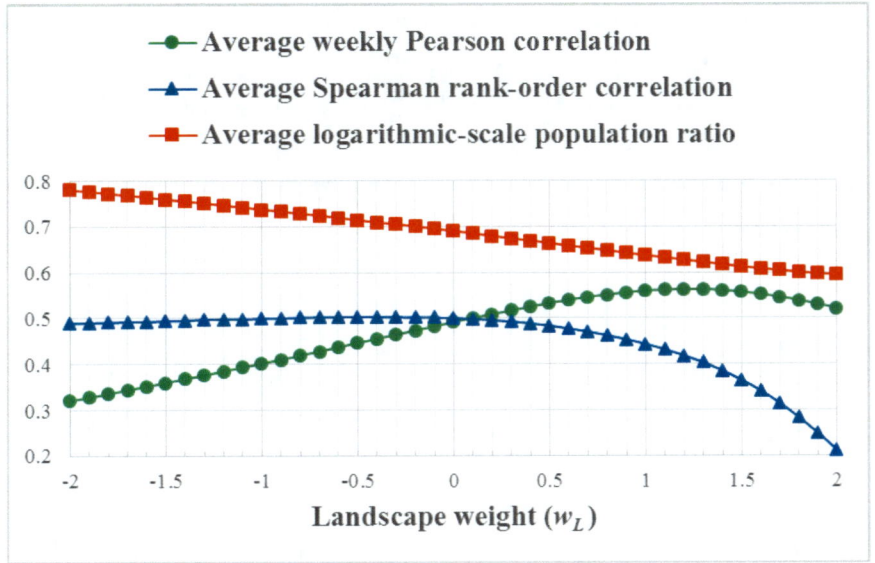

Figure 4. Variations of average of the three metrics for 2004 to 2014 with respect to landscape weight (w_L).

Future Research and Limitations

Using the number of WNV cases among humans in North America to indicate the importance of each specific land cover class for mosquito breeding is likely not the best solution. As such the weight, w_L, of the land cover parameter, L, may not have proper impact to describe the capacity of an environment for mosquito production. This is the primary reason why there is a relatively high number of generated mosquitoes in water regions which have an unknown value of L in the collected dataset. If suitable data regarding the landscape features are available, the land cover parameter (L) could also directly affect the alpha parameter of the birth rate (α_b) as to indicate the environment carrying capacity of female adult mosquitoes. Alternative solutions to quantitatively map each land cover class to a mosquito density descriptor could be crucial future research. Within this context, simple fuzzy rule-based systems could be used to transfer experts' knowledge of preferred land cover by mosquitoes. Such a fuzzy system would consider the proportion of each land cover class present in a mosquito cell, and would then produce one (or more) descriptor(s) for mosquito birth rate or habitat preference. Once the fuzzy system is constructed, all the w_L values or other similar metrics could be pre-calculated for each mosquito cell. Then, the values would be loaded when the simulation is started to boost the performance.

References

[1] Hayes, Edward B., Nicholas Komar, Roger S. Nasci, Susan P. Montgomery, Daniel R. O'Leary, and Grant L. Campbell. "Epidemiology and Transmission Dynamics of West Nile Virus Disease." *Emerging Infectious Diseases* 11 (2005): 1167–73. doi:10.3201/eid1108.050289a.

[2] Colpitts, Tonya M., Michael J. Conway, Ruth R. Montgomery, and Erol Fikrig. "West Nile Virus: Biology, Transmission, and Human Infection." *Clinical Microbiology Reviews* 25 (2012): 635–648. doi:10.1128/CMR.00045-12.

[3] Kramer, Laura D., Linda M. Styer, and Gregory D. Ebel. "A Global Perspective on the Epidemiology of West Nile Virus." *Annual Review of Entomology* 53 (2008): 61–81. doi:10.1146/annurev.ento.53.103106.093258.

[4] Curry, Philip. "Saskatchewan Mosquitoes and West Nile Virus." *Blue Jay* (2004): 104–111.

[5] Kilpatrick, A. Marm, Laura D. Kramer, Scott R. Campbell, E. Oscar Alleyne, Andrew P. Dobson, and Peter Daszak. "West Nile Virus Risk Assessment and the Bridge Vector Paradigm." *Emerging Infectious Diseases* 11 (2005): 425–429. doi:10.3201/eid1103.040364.

[6] Turell, Michael J., M. R. Sardelis, M. L. O'guinn, and D. J. Dohm. "Potential Vectors of West Nile Virus in North America." *Current Topics in Microbiology and Immunology* 267 (2002): 241–52. http://www.ncbi.nlm.nih.gov/pubmed/12082992.

[7] Hamer, Gabriel L., Uriel D. Kitron, Jeffrey D. Brawn, Scott R. Loss, Marilyn O. Ruiz, Tony L. Goldberg, and Edward D. Walker. "Culex pipiens (Diptera: Culicidae): A Bridge Vector of West Nile Virus to Humans." *Journal of Medical Entomology* 45 (2008): 125–8. http://www.ncbi.nlm.nih.gov/pubmed/18283952.

[8] Kilpatrick, A. Marm. "Globalization, Land Use, and the Invasion of West Nile Virus." *Science* 334 (2011): 323–327. doi:10.1126/science.1201010.

[9] Rappole, John H., Bradley W. Compton, Peter Leimgruber, Jamie Robertson, David I. King, and Swen C. Renner. "Modeling Movement of West Nile Virus in the Western Hemisphere." *Vector-Borne Zoonotic Diseases* 6 (2006): 128–139. doi:10.1673/031.007.0501.

[10] Li, Z., J. Hayse, I. Hlohowskyj, K. Smith, and R. Smith. "Agent-based Model for Simulation of West Nile Virus Transmission." *The Agent 2005 Conference on Generative Social Processes, Models, and Mechanisms* (2005): 459–472. http://mysite.science.uottawa.ca/rsmith43/AgentbasedmodelWNV.pdf.

[11] Ward, Michael P., Arlo Raim, Sarah Yaremych-Hamer, Richard Lampman, and Robert J. Novak. "Does the Roosting Behavior of Birds affect Transmission Dynamics of West Nile Virus?" *American Journal of Tropical Medicine and Hygiene* 75 (2006): 350–5. http://www.ncbi.nlm.nih.gov/pubmed/16896147.

[12] Krebs, Bethany L., Tavis K. Anderson, Tony L. Goldberg, Gabriel L. Hamer, Uriel D. Kitron, Christina M. Newman, Marilyn O. Ruiz, Edward D. Walker, and Jeffrey D. Brawn. "Host Group Formation Decreases Exposure to Vector-borne Disease: A Field Experiment in a "Hotspot" of West Nile Virus Transmission." *Proceedings of the Royal Society B: Biological Sciences* 281 (2014). http://rspb.royalsocietypublishing.org/content/281/1796/20141586.

[13] Janousek, William M., Peter P. Marra, and A. Marm Kilpatrick. "Avian Roosting Behavior Influences Vector-Host Interactions for West Nile Virus Hosts." *Parasites and Vectors* 7 (2014): 399. doi:10.1186/1756-3305-7-399.

[14] Chevalier, Véronique, Annelise Tran, and Benoit Durand. "Predictive Modeling of West Nile Virus Transmission Risk in the Mediterranean Basin: How far from Landing?" *International Journal of Environmental Research and Public Health* 11 (2013): 67–90. doi:10.3390/ijerph110100067.

[15] Hamer, Gabriel L., Uriel D. Kitron, Tony L. Goldberg, Jeffrey D. Brawn, Scott R. Loss, Marilyn O. Ruiz, Daniel B. Hayes, and Edward D. Walker. "Host Selection by Culex pipiens Mosquitoes and West Nile Virus Amplification." *American Journal of Tropical Medicine and Hygiene* 80 (2009): 268–278. doi:80/2/268 [pii].

[16] Marm Kilpatrick, A., Peter Daszak, Matthew J. Jones, Peter P. Marra, and Laura D. Kramer. "Host Heterogeneity Dominates West Nile Virus Transmission." *Proceedings of the Royal Society B: Biological Sciences* 273 (2006): 2327–2333. doi:10.1098/rspb.2006.3575.

[17] Hamer, Gabriel L., Luis F. Chaves, Tavis K. Anderson, Uriel D. Kitron, Jeffrey D. Brawn, Marilyn O. Ruiz, Scott R. Loss, Edward D. Walker, and Tony L. Goldberg. "Fine-scale Variation in Vector Host Use and Force of Infection Drive Localized Patterns of West Nile Virus Transmission." *PLoS One* 6 (2011). doi:10.1371/journal.pone.0023767.

[18] Kent, Rebekah, Lara Juliusson, Michael Weissmann, Sara Evans, and Nicholas Komar. "Seasonal Blood-Feeding Behavior of Culex tarsalis (Diptera: Culicidae) in Weld County, Colorado, 2007." *Journal of Medical Entomology* 46 (2009): 380–390. doi:10.1603/033.046.0226.

[19] Molaei, Goudarz, Theodore G. Andreadis, Philip M. Armstrong, Rudy Bueno Jr, James A. Dennett, Susan V. Real, Chris Sargent et al. "Host Feeding Pattern of Culex quinquefasciatus (Diptera: Culicidae) and its Role in Transmission of West Nile Virus in Harris County, Texas." *American Journal of Tropical Medicine and Hygiene* 77 (2007): 73–81. doi:77/1/73 [pii].

[20] Molaei, Goudarz, Robert F. Cummings, Tianyun Su, Philip M. Armstrong, Greg A. Williams, Min-Lee Cheng, James P. Webb, and Theodore G. Andreadis. "Vector-host Interactions Governing Epidemiology of West Nile Virus in Southern California." *American*

Journal of Tropical Medicine and Hygiene 83 (2010): 1269–1282. doi:10.4269/ajtmh.2010.10-0392.

[21] Cooke, William H., Katarzyna Grala, and Robert C. Wallis. "Avian GIS Models Signal Human Risk for West Nile Virus in Mississippi." *International Journal of Health Geographics* 5 (2006): 36. doi:10.1186/1476-072X-5-36.

[22] Paull, Sara H., Daniel E. Horton, Moetasim Ashfaq, Deeksha Rastogi, Laura D. Kramer, Noah S. Diffenbaugh, and A. Marm Kilpatrick. "Drought and Immunity Determine the Intensity of West Nile Virus Epidemics and Climate Change Impacts." *Proceedings of the Royal Society B: Biological Sciences* 284 (2017): 20162078. doi:10.1098/rspb.2016.2078.

[23] Turell, Michael J., David J. Dohm, Michael R. Sardelis, Monica L. O'guinn, Theodore G. Andreadis, and Jamie A. Blow. "An Update on the Potential of North American Mosquitoes (Diptera: Culicidae) to Transmit West Nile Virus." *Journal of Medical Entomology* 42 (2005): 57–62. doi:10.1603/0022-2585(2005)042[0057:AUOTPO]2.0.CO;2.

[24] Barr, A. Ralph. "Occurrence and Distribution of the Culex pipiens Complex." *Bulletin of the World Health Organization* 37 (1967): 293–296.

[25] Apperson, Charles S., Bruce A. Harrison, Thomas R. Unnasch, Hassan K. Hassan, William S. Irby, Harry M. Savage, Stephen E. Aspen et al. "Host-Feeding Habits of *Culex* and Other Mosquitoes (Diptera: Culicidae) in the Borough of Queens in New York City, with Characters and Techniques for Identification of *Culex* Mosquitoes." *Journal of Medical Entomology* 39 (2002): 777–785. doi:10.1603/0022-2585-39.5.777.

[26] Andreadis, Theodore G. "The Contribution of Culex pipiens Complex Mosquitoes to Transmission and Persistence of West Nile Virus in North America." *Journal of the American Mosquito Control Association* 28 (2012): 137–151. doi:10.2987/8756-971X-28.4s.137.

[27] Chen, Chen-Chih, Tasha Epp, Emily Jenkins, Cheryl Waldner, Philip Curry, and Catherine Soos. "Modeling Monthly Variation of Culex tarsalis (Diptera: Culicidae) Abundance and West Nile Virus Infection

Rate in the Canadian Prairies." *International Journal of Environmental Research and Public Health* 10 (2013): 3033–3051. doi:10.3390/ijerph10073033.

[28] Yiannakoulias, Nikolaos W., Donald P. Schopflocher, and Lawrence W. Svenson. "Modelling Geographic Variations in West Nile Virus." *Canadian Journal of Public Health* 97 (2006): 374–378.

[29] Government of Manitoba. *Surveillance for West Nile virus in Manitoba. In: Manitoba Health, Seniors and Active Living.* Accessed April 15, 2015. http://www.gov.mb.ca/health/wnv/stats.html.

[30] Goddard, Laura B., Amy E. Roth, William K. Reisen, and Thomas W. Scott. "Vertical Transmission of West Nile Virus by Three California Culex (Diptera: Culicidae) Species." *Journal of Medical Entomology* 40 (2003): 743–746. doi:10.1603/0022-2585-40.6.743.

[31] Tempelis, C. H., W. C. Reeves, R. E. Bellamy, and M. F. Lofy. "A Three-Year Study of the Feeding Habits of Culex tarsalis in Kern County, California." *American Journal fo Tropical Medicine and Hygiene* 14 (1965): 170–177. doi:10.4269/ajtmh.1965.14.170.

[32] Reisen, W. "The Western Encephalitis Mosquito, Culex tarsalis." *Wing Beats* 4 (1993): 16. http://www-rci.rutgers.edu/~insects/sp6.htm.

[33] North Dakota Grand Forks Public Health. *Local Mosquito Species.* Accessed April 21, 2015. http://www.gfmosquito.com/local-mosquito-species/.

[34] American Mosquito Control Association. *Mosquito Life Cycle.* Accessed April 15, 2015. http://www.mosquito.org/life-cycle. Archived at: http://www.webcitation.org/6iJntDZde.

[35] Hearle, Eric. *The Mosquitoes of the Lower Fraser Valley, British Columbia, and their Control.* Ottawa: 1926. https://www.cabdirect.org/cabdirect/abstract/19271000059.

[36] McLintock, J. "The Mosquitoes of the Greater Winnipeg Area." *Canadian Entomology* 76 (1944) 89–104. doi:10.4039/Ent7689-5.

[37] Abdelrazec, Ahmed, and Abba B. Gumel. "Mathematical Assessment of the Role of Temperature and Rainfall on Mosquito Population Dynamics." *Journal of Mathematical Biology* 42 (2016). doi:10.1007/s00285-016-1054-9.

[38] Okuneye, Kamaldeen, and Abba B. Gumel. "Analysis of a Temperature- and Rainfall-dependent Model for Malaria Transmission Dynamics." *Mathematical Biosciences* 2016. doi:10.1016/j.mbs.2016.03.013.

[39] Government of Manitoba. *Land Use / Land Cover, Manitoba Land Initiative.* Accessed September 29, 2015. http://mli2.gov.mb.ca/landuse/index.html.

[40] Bowden, Sarah E., Krisztian Magori, and John M. Drake. Regional Differences in the Association Between Land Cover and West Nile Virus Disease Incidence in Humans in the United States." *American Journal of Tropical Medicine and Hygiene* 84 (2011): 234–238. doi:10.4269/ajtmh.2011.10-0134.

[41] Anderson, James R. "A Land Use and Land Cover Classification System for Use with Remote Sensor Data." *Professional Paper* 964 (1976).

[42] Komar, Nicholas, Stanley Langevin, Steven Hinten, Nicole Nemeth, Eric Edwards, Danielle Hettler, Brent Davis, Richard Bowen, and Michel Bunning. "Experimental Infection of North American Birds with the New York 1999 Strain of West Nile Virus." *Emerging Infectious Diseases* 9 (2003): 311–322. doi:10.3201/eid0903.020628.

[43] Kilpatrick, A. Marm, Shannon L. LaDeau, and Peter P. Marra. "Ecology of West Nile Virus Tansmission and its Impact on Birds in the Western Hemisphere." *Auk* 124 (2007): 1121–1136. doi:10.1642/0004-8038(2007)124[1121:EOWNVT]2.0.CO;2.

[44] Thiemann, Tara C., Sarah S. Wheeler, Christopher M. Barker, and William K. Reisen. "Mosquito Host Selection Varies Seasonally with Host Availability and Mosquito Density." *PLoS Neglected Tropical Diseases* 5 (2011): e1452. doi:10.1371/journal.pntd.0001452.

[45] Reisen, William K., Hugh D. Lothrop, and Tara Thiemann. "Host Selection Patterns of Culex tarsalis (Diptera: Culicidae) at Wetlands near the Salton Sea, Coachella Valley, California, 1998-2002." *Journal of Medical Entolomology* 50 (2013): 1071–6. http://www.pubmedcentral.nih.gov/articlerender.fcgi?artid=3918163&tool=pmcentrez&rendertype=abstract.

[46] Campbell, Rebecca, Tara C. Thiemann, Debra Lemenager, and William K. Reisen. "Host-Selection Patterns of Culex tarsalis (Diptera : Culicidae) Determine the Spatial Heterogeneity of West Nile Virus Enzootic Activity in Northern California." *Journal of Medical Entomology* 50 (2013): 1303–9. doi:10.1603/me13089.

[47] Komar, Nicholas. "West Nile Virus: Epidemiology and Ecology in North America." *Advances in Virus Research* 61 (2003): 185–234. doi:10.1016/S0065-3527(03)61005-5.

[48] Clements, A. N. *The Biology of Mosquitoes: Sensory Reception and Behaviour*. New York: Chapman & Hall, 1992.

[49] Bargaoui, Ramzi, Sylvie Lecollinet, and Renaud Lancelot. "Mapping the Serological Prevalence Rate of West Nile Fever in Equids, Tunisia." *Transboundary and Emerging Diseases* 62 (2015): 55–66. doi:10.1111/tbed.12077.

[50] Ward, Michael P. "Equine West Nile Virus Disease Occurrence and the Normalized Difference Vegetation Index." *Preventive Veterinary Medicine* 88 (2009): 205–12. doi:10.1016/j.prevetmed.2008.10.003.

[51] Prairie Pest Monitoring Network. *Drought Watch - Map Archive. In: Agriculture and Agri-Food Canada*. http://www.agr.gc.ca/DW-GS/historical-historiques.jspx?lang=eng&jsEnabled=true.

[52] Allen, Jon C. "A Modified Sine Wave Method for Calculating Degree Days." *Environmental Entomology* 5 (1976).

[53] Reisen, William K., Ying Fang, and Vincent M. Martinez. "Effects of Temperature on the Transmission of West Nile Virus by Culex tarsalis (Diptera: Culicidae)." *Journal of Medical Entomology* 43 (2006): 309–317. doi:10.1603/0022-2585(2006)043[0309:eotott]2.0.co;2.

[54] Zou, Li, Scott N. Miller, and Edward T. Schmidtmann. "A GIS Tool to Estimate West Nile Virus Risk Based on a Degree-day Model." *Environmental Monitoring and Assessment* 129 (2007): 413–420. doi:10.1007/s10661-006-9373-8.

In: West Nile Virus
Editor: Marinke van Verseveld

ISBN: 978-1-53616-589-0
© 2019 Nova Science Publishers, Inc.

Chapter 2

RECOMBINANT ENVELOPE DOMAIN III PROTEIN OF WEST NILE VIRUS: RECENT DEVELOPMENTS AND APPLICATIONS

Nagesh K. Tripathi[*] *and Ambuj Shrivastava*
Defence Research and Development Establishment, Gwalior, India

ABSTRACT

West Nile virus (WNV), a mosquito-borne, single-stranded, positive-sense flavivirus, has been linked to acute viral encephalitis and neurological sequelae. Currently neither any antiviral drugs nor any vaccines are licensed for human use. Recent developments on recombinant proteins have paved the way to produce various viral proteins which have potential to be used as diagnostic or vaccine candidates. These recombinant viral proteins are generally produced in microbial and higher expression host systems such as bacteria, insect cells, and transgenic plants. The genome of West Nile virus encodes three structural proteins [capsid (C) protein, pre-membrane (prM) protein and envelope (E) protein) and seven non-structural (NS1, NS2A, NS2B, NS3, NS4A, NS4B, NS5) proteins. The envelope (E) protein has three domains (Domain I, II and III) and it

---

[*] Corresponding Author's E-mail:tripathink@gmail.com;tripathink@drde.drdo.in.

mediates viral binding to cellular receptors and has fusogenic property with the host cell membrane. The domain III (DIII) of E protein contains the neutralizing epitopes that induce strong host antibody responses and provide protective immunity. Due to these reasons, the domain III of E protein can be utilized as recombinant protein vaccine candidate as well as diagnostic intermediate for WNV. In this chapter, we summarize about the the envelope domain III (EDIII) protein, its production using various host systems and applications in the development of WNV vaccines and diagnostics.

Keywords: West Nile virus, recombinant protein, envelope domain III, vaccine

INTRODUCTION

West Nile virus (WNV) of the family *Flaviviridae*, genus *Flavivirus* has emerged as an increasingly important viral pathogen for humans and domestic animals. WNV is a small enveloped virus having a diameter of 50 nm (Martín-Acebes and Saiz 2012). Symptoms of West Nile fever includes a mild illness progressing to a severe illness, sudden onset, headache, malaise, fever, myalgia, chills, vomiting, rash, fatigue, and eye pain (Petersen et al. 2013). There is no licensed vaccine for human available till date for WNV; however, various vaccine candidates are under different pre-clinical and clinical phases. The vaccine candidates intended for human include inactivated virus, live attenuated virus, DNA, virus vectored and recombinant protein vaccines. The recombinant protein vaccine candidates include E and EDIII proteins (Bonafé et al. 2009; Chu et al. 2007; Martina et al. 2008; Watts et al. 2007). These proteins were successfully expressed using *E. coli* (Tan et al. 2010; Chu et al. 2007; Tripathi et al. 2018a), insect cells (Bonafé et al. 2009) and transgenic plants (He et al. 2014; Chen 2015; Lai et al. 2018). The recombinant proteins are generally expressed in prokaryotic and eukaryotic hosts employing genetic engineering tools. In the present review, we describe recent developments in recombinant West Nile virus EDIII protein.

WNV EDIII Protein, Its Expression and Purification

West Nile virus consists of a nucleocapsid surrounded by an envelope layer. The genome of WNV is a positive-sense RNA (~10.7 kilobase) consisting of a single open reading frame (ORF). This ORF translates into a single polyprotein which is further cleaved with the help of proteases of both host cell and virus. This leads to the production of three structural protens viz. capsid (C), precursor membrane (prM), and envelope (E) and seven non-structural proteins viz. NS1, NS2A, NS2B, NS3, NS4A, NS4B, and NS5 (Martín-Acebes and Saiz 2012; Londono-Renteria and Colpitts 2016; Brinton 2013). The envelope functions as a transmembrane protein which is attached to the lipid envelope by a C-terminal α-helical hairpin. This protein is most important immunogen and contains the crucial epitopes for eliciting most of the neutralizing antibodies (Beasley 2005). X-ray crystallography showed that it is organized in three domains): DI, DII are responsible for fusion of virus with the cell due to a hydrophobic peptide called fusion loop whereas DIII is an immunoglobulin-like domain. DII is responsible for homodimerization of the protein on the surface of the virion (Nybakken et al. 2006; Kanai et al. 2006). DIII is mainly responsible for receptor binding and harbours many epitopes leading to the induction of neutralizing antibodies (Martín-Acebes and Saiz 2012). Various studies have been carried out using EDIII proteins of West Nile virus for the development of vaccines (Chu et al. 2007; Tan et al. 2010; Tripathi et al. 2018a). Thus, this protein can be used in the development of recombinant subunit vaccines against West Nile virus infection.

The choice of expression systems determines critical aspects of recombinant proteins based vaccine production, including product yield, product quality, scale-up, timelines, and cost of products (Tripathi and Shrivastava 2018; Tripathi 2016). Most of the recombinant WNV proteins for prophylactic or diagnostic use are expressed in *E. coli*, insect cells and transgenic plants. *E. coli* is the most preferred prokaryotic expression system for production of recombinant proteins as it grows rapidly on inexpensive substrates. Its genetics is well characterized and understood (Tripathi 2016). For the expression of WNV EDIII proteins, the EDIII gene is first cloned into expression vectors. Further, the *E. coli* is transformed with the recombinant plasmids for recombinant EDIII protein expression. Mostly the protein expression is induced by chemical inducer isopropyl-β-D-thiogalactoside at mid-log phase during cultivation (Tan et al. 2010). Small scale expression and process optimization are generally carried out using shake flask cultures. For scale up production of EDIII proteins, bioreactor cultures are used in batch and fed-batch mode to improve the volumetric and specific yield. The most important optimization parameters for the high yield expression of recombinant proteins include culture media, cultivation temperature, induction time, inducer concentration and pH. For small scale expression of recombinant EDIII proteins, the shake flask culture is commonly used. During the scale-up process, bioreactor cultures of different scale are generally used to increase the protein yield (Tripathi et al. 2018a). After successful expression of recombinant proteins, there is a need to purify this protein for further use in vaccine development studies. For easy purification of this protein, generally the recombinant protein is expressed as a fusin protein such as the hexahistidine tag (Tan et al. 2010). It allows ease of purification using immobilized metal-ion affinity chromatography (IMAC). For the purification of recombinant EDIII proteins expressed in inclusion bodies, the cell pellet is first lysed using sonication and then IBs are solubilized using denaturants such as Urea. The clear solubilized solution after centrifugation is then loaded onto the IMAC column for final purification. Refolding or renaturation of this IBs expressed protein is necessary to obtain biologically active protein for vaccine studies. For soluble expression, protein is purified from clear lysate using IMAC. After initial purification using IMAC, the purity level of EDIII proteins can be further increased by ion exchange or size exclusion chromatography (Tripathi et al. 2018a). Insect cells are also utilized as a host for recombinant WNV protein expression. In this expression system the recombinant proteins are secreted in the serum free media and easily purified with minimum number of steps. For the expression of recombinant WNV proteins in insect cells, the respective gene is cloned and transfected into *Drosophila* S2 cells.

Recombinant protein is purified from the cell culture supernatant by ion-exchange chromatography followed by size-exclusion chromatography (Ledizet et al. 2005). Plant biotechnology also plays a crucial role in production of vaccines, antigens and subunits by using genetic modification (Sohrab et al. 2017). Transgenic plants offer high yield and easy scale up for recombinant protein production. Absence of potentially harmful pathogens of concern to humans and near-normal glycosylation occurs in this system (Yap and Smith 2010). Transgenic plants is generally produced by inserting the gene of interest into a virus e.g., Tobacco Mosaic Virus (TMV), that is found in plants or by inserting the desired gene directly into the plant DNA using gene gun technology. Plant expression vectors for WNV EDIII are agroinfiltrated into leaves of *N. benthamiana* plants. Leaves are harvested 4 days post agroinfiltration (dpi) and EDIII protein is extracted and purified with IMAC (He et al. 2014; Lai et al. 2018).

RECOMBINANT EDIII PROTEIN IN DIAGNOSIS OF WNV INFECTION

WNV has emerged as an important viral pathogen for human and animal disease worldwide. To control the spread of the WNV disease, early detection of WNV infection is necessary. The current diagnosis of WNV disease is based on serology using ELISA, virus isolation using cell culture and RNA detection by molecular assays (De Filette et al. 2012; Petersen et al. 2013; Barzon et al. 2015). Serological assays such as antibody capture ELISA (MAC-ELISA) and indirect ELISA are mostly used as surveillance tool to detect WNV infections in patient serum and CSF samples due to ease of use and good sensitivity. IgG avidity testing is most useful to differentiate between acute and past WNV infection. WNV lateral flow assay was also developed based on recombinant E protein and anti-E monoclonal antibody for detection of anti-human IgM antibody. NS1 antigen capture ELISA is also available for detection of WNV NS1 antigen in patient serum samples (Petersen et al. 2013; Barzon et al. 2015). Recombinant WNV EDIII protein-based ELISA has been developed and evaluated. In a study, *E. coli* expressed EDIII of the WNV could clearly differentiate antibody responses to WNV from those against other related flaviviruses in indirect ELISA (Beasley et al. 2004). In another study, EDIII of WNV was bacterially expressed and purified. An ELISA with this antigen established that this antigen may be a potentially useful tool for serologic diagnosis of WNV infections (Chávez et al. 2013). A monoclonal antibody (1D11), that recognizes an epitope in the EDIII of WNV, was used in immunochromatographic assay and was able to detect all WNV strains, and did not cross-react with other non-WNV arboviruses (Rebollo et al. 2018).

WNV Vaccine Development and Current Status

Currently, there is no licensed human vaccine against WNV. However, various licensed vaccines are available against WNV for veterinary use in the market (Chen 2015; Amanna and Slifka 2014; Ulbert 2019).Various approaches have been used for the development of human vaccine candidates against WNV (Iyer and Kousoulas 2013; Ulbert and Magnusson 2014; Chen 2015; Ulbert 2019; Krol et al. 2019; Scherwitzl et al. 2017). Among all the vaccine candidates, the frontrunner is ChimeriVax which is a live attenuated vaccine. In this vaccine candidate, prM and E genes of Yellow Fever Virus (YF-17D) have been replaced by those of the WNV NY99 strain, thus expressing WNV antigens in a YF 17D backbone. This vaccine has completed Phase II clinical trials. ChimeriVax-WN01 was commercialized as a veterinary vaccine. Further, ChimeriVax-WN02 vaccine was developed for human use by engineering three mutations in the E gene to reduce neurovirulence (Dayan et al. 2013; G. H. Dayan et al. 2012). Another Chimeric vaccine (WN/DEN4Δ30) has also been developed and consists of the WNV prM and E genes inserted into an attenuated dengue virus type 4 vaccine strain. This vaccine candidate has completed two phase I clinical trials (Pierce et al. 2017; Durbin et al. 2013). An inactivated WNV vaccine (HydroVax-001) was also developed using a H_2O_2 based process. In 2015, HydroVax-001 also entered in phase I clinical trial (Woods et al.

2019). In a recent study, HydroVax-II was also developed utilizing reduced concentrations of H_2O_2 together with copper complexed methisazone (MZ-antiviral compound,). This study resulted in rapid virus inactivation and 130-fold higher WNV-specific neutralizing antibody response in comparision to that of the first generation (H_2O_2 only vaccine approach) and conferred 100% protection against lethal WNV infection (Quintel et al. 2019). A DNA plasmid vaccine (VRC302) expressing the WNV proteins prM and E was also developed. During the Phase I clinical trial, this vaccine showed the safety and immunogenicity in humans. Further, promoter was modified to increase the immunogenicity and also tested during a second phase I clinical trial (VRC-303) which resulted in induction of T cell response of greater magnitude in comparison to VRC-302 (Ledgerwood et al. 2011; Martin et al. 2007). Recombinant subunit vaccine candidate (WN-80E) was also developed. This WN-80E was produced by expression of soluble form of the E protein of WNV without the transmembrane domain in *Drosophila melanogaster* insect cells. This vaccine was also tested in a phase I trial and showed that the vaccine was well tolerated (Coller et al. 2012; Chen 2015; Amanna and Slifka 2014). The list of vaccine candidates for WNV which have undergone various phases of clinical trials is shown in Table 1.

Researchers also studied the protection potential of *E. coli* expressed E-ectodomain of WNV protein and established that this protein demonstrated protection in animal models with high antigen doses. The expression of E ectodomain of WNV as a recombinant thioredoxin fusion protein was carried out in *E.coli*. This protein was formulated with FCA and immunized in mice model. This study reported that this vaccine candidate provided protection in a WNV challenge model. Further, human serum antibodies (WNV-infected individuals previously) were able to recognize the recombinant E protein (Wang et al. 2001). In another study, recombinant WNV E protein (NY 99 strain) was expressed in *E. coli* and purified after oxidative refolding. This protein was mixed with the particulate *Quillaja saponaria*, a saponin-based adjuvant. This adjuvant induced a broader immune response (Th1 and Th2), in comparison to antigen alone or antigen formulated with other adjuvants (Oliphant et al. 2007; Magnusson et al. 2014; Ulbert and Magnusson 2014).

Table 1. Status of WNV vaccines candidates in clinical trials

Vaccine candidate	Type	Approach of the study	Current status	References
rWNV/DEN4Δ30 (NIAID)	Live attenuated	Dengue virus type 4 backbone expressing West Nile virus prM and envelope	Phase I	(Durbin et al. 2013; Pierce et al. 2017)
ChimeriVax-WN02 (Sanofi Pasteur)	Live attenuated	Yellow Fever virus 17D backbone expressing West Nile virus prM and envelope	Phase II	(Dayan et al. 2012; Dayan et al. 2013)
HydroVax-001 (Oregon Health and Science University/NIAID)	Inactivated using Hydrogen peroxide	West Nile virus	Phase I	(Woods et al. 2019)
HBV-002 (Hawaii Biotech)	Recombinant subunit	West Nile virus recombinant truncated E protein	Phase I	(Coller et al. 2012)
VRC 302/VRC 303 (Vial/NIAID)	DNA	Plasmid DNA expressing West Nile virus prM-envelope	Phase I	(Ledgerwood et al. 2011)
Inactivated WNV	Inactivated using formaldehyde	West Nile virus strain NY99	Phase I/II	(Barrett et al. 2017)

Chen 2015; Amanna and Slifka 2014; Scherwitzl et al. 2017; Ulbert 2019

A truncated form of WNV E protein was produced in *Drosophila* S2 cells and this protein was studied for immunogenicity in mice and horses. Recombinant E protein combined with aluminum hydroxide adjuvant resulted in high-titer antibodies in mice and horses. Immunized mice were protected upon challenge study. Further, the sera from immunized horses when administered to naïve mice provided protection against a lethal WNV (Ledizet et al. 2005). A recombinant truncated WNV E protein antigen was produced using *expres*SF+ insect cell line via baculovirus infection. This protein was evaluated for immunogenicity and protective efficacy in mouse and hamster using aluminum hydroxide. The results of this study established that insectcell produced protein induced humoral immunity that can protect against WNV infection (Bonafé et al. 2009). In a study, insect cells expressed and purified nonstructural 1 protein was immunized in hamsters followed by lethal WNV challenge. This NS1 vaccine could reduce viremia and moderately increase survival rates (87% survival) in comparison to control animals (47% survival). The study also reported the vaccine potential of E protein expressed using insect cells. The adjuvant used for this study was ISCOMATRIX® adjuvant (Watts et al. 2007; Lieberman et al. 2007).

Various studies were also carried out to develop VLPs based WNV vaccine candidates (Krol et al. 2019). Co-expression of prM and E often results into the assembly of VLPs and these VLPs have many immunogenic properties similar to that of the native virions (Ohtaki et al. 2010). In a study, prM/E or C, prM and E proteins (C-prM/E) VLPs were generated in insect cells (Sf9) by the co-expression of prM and E proteins. These VLPs induced protective immunity in mice (Qiao et al. 2004). In another study, lineage 1 WNV prM-E VLP was produced from mammalian cell. A single dose of lineage 1 WNV prM-E VLPs was able to protect mice against a lethal challenge of WNV (both lineage 1 and 2). This study established that VLPs based vaccines have an edge over the individual subunit vaccines (Merino-Ramos et al. 2014). The prM-E VLPs was succesfully produced transiently using a Herpes Simplex Virus replication defective vector. Immunization of mice with the d106-WNV recombinant vector elicited a specific anti-WNV IgG response (Taylor et al. 2016). VLP-based WNV vaccine was also evaluated using AP205 (RNA bacteriophage). For this purpose, EDII protein was either chemically cross-linked to VLPs (Spohn et al. 2010) or genetically fused to coat protein of AP205 (Cielens et al. 2014). In both cases, chimeric VLPs with or without different adjuvants were highly immunogenic in mice (Krol et al. 2019). In another study, HBcAg-EDIII chimeric VLPs that display the EDIII epitopes on its surface were produced using *N. benthamiana*. Immunization of a single dose (25 µg) of HBcAg-EDIII VLPs in mice induced strong EDIII-specific B and T-cell responses that are greater than that of the non-fused EDIII antigen (Chen 2015).

Various efforts were also made to develop a virus vectored WNV vaccine candidates based on a Canarypox viral vector expressing prM and E proteins, Vesicular Stomatitis Virus vector and lentiviral vectors expressing E protein (Iyer et al. 2009; Coutant et al. 2008; Brandler and Tangy 2013; Chen 2015). WNV E glycoprotein was expressed using a Vesicular Stomatitis Virus and generated strong humoral and cellular immunity.

Further, it also provided protection in mice from lethal WNV challenge (Iyer et al. 2009). The soluble form of the E glycoprotein from the ISR98 WNV strain was also expressed using a lentiviral HIV1-TRIP vector. This protein induced a durable protective and sterilizing humoral immune response (Iglesias et al. 2006). Due to safety concerns, a similar, but non-integrative, lentiviral vector was further produced that elicited a robust B-cell response. It was also able to fully protect mice from lethal WNV challenge (Coutant et al. 2008).

In another study, the CD16 ectodomain of CD16-RIgE was replaced by EDIII of WNV Kunjin (WNV^{Kun}). In Sf9 insect cells, the recombinant Pr55Gag^{HIV} was efficiently self-assembled into VLPs. Substitution of the CD16 ectodomain by the EDIII allowed the display of EDIII at the surface of the VLPs and thereby inducing neutralizing antibody response in mice (Brandler and Tangy 2013; Chua et al. 2013).

DNA vaccine expressing the domain III (DIII) region of the Envelope protein has been developed and tested in animal model (Ramanathan et al. 2009). In efforts to develop a chimeric peptide vaccine for WNV, a continuous B-cell epitope derived from WNV EDIII (named Ep15) was fused to HSP60 p458 peptide as the carrier. Immunization of mice was carried out using this chimeric peptide and provided protection against three different WNV strains (Gershoni-Yahalom et al. 2010).

RECOMBINANT WNV EDIII PROTEIN AS SUBUNIT VACCINE CANDIDATES

The EDIII of flaviviruses harbours the receptor binding epitopes and is responsible for generation of virus-neutralizing antibodies. This EDIII protein has been targeted as an attractive vaccine candidate for the development of recombinant protein vaccines (Diamond et al. 2008; Pierson et al. 2008; Brandler and Tangy 2013; Tripathi et al. 2018b). Various studies reported that recombinant EDIII protein of WNV can elicit immune responses that confer protection in mice against WNV challenge when used with various adjuvants (Brandler and Tangy 2013; Chen 2015; Amanna and Slifka 2014). In a study, recombinant WNV EDIII protein was expressed, purified and refolded. Purified EDIII protein of WNV blocked entry of WNV into Vero cells and C6/36 cells. In plaque neutralization assay, mice serum generated against EDIII protein inhibited infection with WNV (Chu et al. 2005). In a study, *E. coli* expressed and purified EDIII protein of WNV was evaluated in mice. This study resulted in induction of both IgG1 and IgG2a anti-EDIII antibodies indicating a strong Th1 response.

Table 2. Recombinant WNV EDIII protein based vaccine candidates

Vaccine candidate	Expression system	Approach of the study	Animal model	Summarised results	References
WNV EDIII	*E. coli*	West Nile virus envelope domain III protein expressed in *E. coli*	Mice	Inhibited West Nile virus entry into Vero cells and C6/36 cells; Anti-EDIII antibody inhibited infection with West Nile virus	(Chu et al. 2005)
WNV EDIII	*E. coli*	West Nile virus envelope domain III protein expressed in *E. coli*	Mice	CpG-DNA adjuvented EDIII generated high titer of neutralizing antibodies and Th1 immune response	(Chu et al. 2007)
WNV EDIII-STF2Δ	*E. coli*	West Nile virus envelope domain III protein fused to a modified version of bacterial flagellin (STF2Δ) and expressed in *E. coli*	Mice	Induced neutralizing antibodies and protected mice against West Nile virus challenge	(McDonald et al. 2007)
WNV EDIII	*E. coli*	West Nile virus envelope domain III protein expressed in *E. coli*	Mice	Induced high neutralizing antibody titer, provided protection against lethal West Nile virus infection and provided partial protection against lethal JE virus infection	(Martina et al. 2008)
WNV EDIII	*E. coli*	West Nile virus envelope domain III protein expressed in *E. coli*	Mice	Generated EDIII specific antibodies and neutralizing antibodies	(Tan et al. 2010)

Table 2. (Continued)

Vaccine candidate	Expression system	Approach of the study	Animal model	Summarised results	References
WNV EDIII	*E. coli*	West Nile virus envelope domain III protein expressed in *E. coli*	Mice	Less effective in inducing neutralizing antibodies titer than E ectodomain or inactivated complete virions	(Zlatkovic et al. 2011)
WNV EDIII	*E. coli*	West Nile virus envelope domain III protein expressed in *E. coli*	Horse	Immunization of EDIII protein with CD40L adjuvant exhibited significantly stronger neutralizing activity and stimulated CD8+T cells	(Liu et al. 2017)
WNV EDIII	*E. coli*	West Nile virus envelope domain III protein expressed in *E. coli*	Rabbit	Generated EDIII specific antibodies and neutralizing antibodies	(Tripathi et al. 2018a)
WNV EDIII	Insect larvae	West Nile virus envelope domain III protein expressed in insect larvae	Mice	Elicited high antibodies titer and neutralized viral infectivity in cell culture and in suckling mice	(Alonso-Padilla et al. 2011)
WNV EDIII	*Nicotiana benthamiana*	West Nile virus envelope domain III protein expressed in transgenic plant *Nicotiana benthamiana*	Mice	Produced potent systemic response in mice	(He et al. 2014)
WNV EDIII	*Nicotiana benthamiana*	West Nile virus envelope domain III protein expressed in transgenic plant	Mice	Evoked antigen-specific both cellular and humoral immune response as well as induce neutralizing antibodies and provided protection against a lethal challenge of West Nile virus infection in mice	(Lai et al. 2018)

These antibodies conferred protection in neonatal mice against cerebral WNV infection. CpG DNA was used as adjuvant here (Chu et al. 2007). In another study, the EDIII protein was expressed in *E. coli* as a fusion protein with bacterial protein flagellin (STF2Δ). This fusion protein was evaluated in mice and gave rise to WNV neutralizing antibodies and protected mice against a WNV challenge (McDonald et al. 2007). The immunogenicity of

EDIII of WNV expressed in bacteria was studied in C57BL/6 mice. It elicited higher titer of neutralizing antibody and also provided protection in mice from lethal WNV challenge (Martina et al. 2008). *E. coli* expressed and affinity membrane chromatography purified recombinant DIII (rDIII) antigen of WNV was also used for vaccine development study. Immunogenicity of purified EDIII protein was demonstrated by its potential to elicit EDIII specific antibodies in mice that could inhibit the WNV (Tan et al. 2010). In a study, it was also reported that the *E. coli* expressed EDIII protein induced about 15-fold lower titer of neutralizing antibodies than those elicited by the whole virion. However, EDIII was found to be an attractive boosting immunogen (Zlatkovic et al. 2011). A chimeric fusion of the non-toxic cholera toxin (CT) CTA2/B domains to DIII was constructed. The DIII-CTA$_2$/B chimera was expressed in *E. coli* and was evaluated as a novel mucosal WNV vaccine. Mice were immunized intranasally with DIII-CTA2/B, DIII, DIII mixed with CTA2/B, or CTA2/B control, followed by booster dose at 10 day. The mucosal immunization with DIII-CTA2/B resulted in induction of significant DIII-specific humoral immunity (Tinker et al. 2014). In a study, synthetic and supramolecular peptide hydrogels adjuvants with the *E. coli* expressed EDIII of WNV was immunized in mice and the immunogenicity was compared with EDIII with alum adjuvant. The peptide hydrogel formulated protein induced stronger antibody responses and provided protection against WNV challenge (Friedrich et al. 2016). A recombinant vaccine containing WNV EDIII protein I fused in-frame with equine CD40 ligand was expressed in *E. coli* and evaluated in horses. Animals immunized with the EDIII-CD40L protein (with or without TiterMax) resulted in higher neutralization antibodies (Liu et al. 2017). The EDIII of WNV was also produced in *E. coli* using bioreactor by batch and fed-batch process, and purified using affinity and ion exchange chromatography. The purified protein induced EDIII specific antibodies in rabbits and the antibodies were able to neutralize WNV *in vitro* (Tripathi et al. 2018a).

WNV E and WNV EDIII protein were also expressed using insect larvae and used for immunization in mice. The partially purified (E and EDIII) proteins induced higher titer of neutralizing antibodies that inhibited WNV in cell culture and in suckling mice. Upon challenge with WNV NY99, all immunized mice were fully protected (Alonso-Padilla et al. 2011).

Recombinant EDIII protein of WNV was also successfully expressed in transgenic plants for vaccine development studies (Lai et al. 2018; Chen 2015). In a study, EDIII protein of WNV was transiently expressed in in three subcellular compartments in leaves of *N. benthamiana*. EDIII protein was expressed at much higher levels in endoplasmic reticulum (ER) than the chloroplast or the cytosol. Plant ER-derived EDIII was soluble and easily purified to more than 95%. Further, this purified EDIII protein was immunised in mice and it elicited a potent systemic response (He et al. 2014). In another study, the potency of a plant expressed EDIII was studied *in vivo* to study protective immunity against WNV infection. This EDIII vaccine candidate elicited EDIII specific both cellular and humoral immune responses. Furthermore, passive immunization of anti-EDIII mouse serum conferred full protection against a lethal WNV challenge in mice. It was also reported that EDIII specific antibodies did not enhance Zika virus and Dengue virus infection in Fc gamma receptor expressing cells. This eliminates the risk of WNV vaccines in inducing cross-reactive antibodies and sensitizing vaccines to antibody dependent enhancement (ADE) phenomenon (Lai et al. 2018). The list of various recombinant WNV envelope domain III protein based vaccine candidates produced using different host systems is shown in Table 2.

CONCLUSION

The worldwide burden of West Nile virus is growing at an alarming rate till a licensed efficacious vaccine against West Nile virus is developed for human. Different vaccine candidates for West Nile virus are at different stages of clinical trials based on various strategies. These include inactivated virus, live attenuated virus, recombinant proteins, DNA, VLPs and virus vectored West Nile virus vaccines. An in-depth understanding of both the virus and human's immunological interactions is warranted for the development of a successful West Nile virus vaccine. Recent progress on recombinant proteins based West Nile virus vaccines using various strategies viz. fusion protein, novel adjuvants, different hosts and VLPs development will provide path for the development of fully efficacious vaccine against West Nile virus. Recombinant protein based vaccines is superior in terms of biohazard issue being non-infectious, easy to produce and scale up and can be cost-effective. Therefore, the recombinant protein vaccines may become promising substitute in comparison to live attenuated/killed vaccines in the future.

REFERENCES

Alonso-Padilla, Julio, Nereida Jiménez de Oya, Ana-Belén Blázquez, Estela Escribano-Romero, José M. Escribano, and Juan-Carlos Saiz. 2011. "Recombinant West Nile Virus Envelope Protein E and Domain III Expressed in Insect Larvae Protects Mice against West Nile Disease." *Vaccine* 29 (9): 1830–35. https://doi.org/10.1016/j.vaccine.2010.12.081.

Amanna, Ian J, and Mark K Slifka. 2014. "Current Trends in West Nile Virus Vaccine Development." *Expert Review of Vaccines* 13 (5): 589–608. https://doi.org/10.1586/14760584.2014.906309.

Barrett, P. Noel, Sara J. Terpening, Doris Snow, Ronald R. Cobb, and Otfried Kistner. 2017. "Vero Cell Technology for Rapid Development of Inactivated Whole Virus Vaccines for Emerging Viral Diseases." *Expert Review of Vaccines* 16 (9): 883–94. https://doi.org/10.1080/14760584.2017.1357471.

Barzon, Luisa, Monia Pacenti, Sebastian Ulbert, and Giorgio Palù. 2015. "Latest Developments and Challenges in the Diagnosis of Human West Nile Virus Infection." *Expert Review of Anti-Infective Therapy* 13 (3): 327–42. https://doi.org/10.1586/14787210.2015.1007044.

Beasley, David. 2005. "Recent Advances in the Molecular Biology of West Nile Virus." *Current Molecular Medicine* 5 (8): 835–50. https://doi.org/10.2174/156652405774962272.

Beasley, David W C, Michael R Holbrook, Amelia P A Travassos Da Rosa, Lark Coffey, Anne-Sophie Carrara, Kathrine Phillippi-Falkenstein, Rudolf P Bohm, et al. 2004. "Use of a Recombinant Envelope Protein Subunit Antigen for Specific Serological Diagnosis of West Nile Virus Infection." *Journal of Clinical Microbiology* 42 (6): 2759–65. https://doi.org/10.1128/JCM.42.6.2759-2765.2004.

Bonafé, Nathalie, Joseph A Rininger, Richard G Chubet, Harald G Foellmer, Stacey Fader, John F Anderson, Sandra L Bushmich, et al. 2009. "A Recombinant West Nile Virus Envelope Protein Vaccine Candidate Produced in Spodoptera Frugiperda ExpresSF+ Cells." *Vaccine* 27 (2): 213–22. https://doi.org/10.1016/j.vaccine.2008.10.046.

Brandler, Samantha, and Frederic Tangy. 2013. "Vaccines in Development against West Nile Virus." *Viruses* 5 (10): 2384–2409. https://doi.org/10.3390/v5102384.

Brinton, Margo. 2013. "Replication Cycle and Molecular Biology of the West Nile Virus." *Viruses* 6 (1): 13–53. https://doi.org/10.3390/v6010013.

Chávez, Juliana Helena, Vinicius Pinho dos Reis, Jaqueline Raymondi Silva, Helen Julie Laure, José Cesar Rosa, Benedito Antônio Lopes da Fonseca, and Luiz Tadeu Moraes Figueiredo. 2013. "Production and Diagnostic Application of Recombinant Domain III of West Nile Envelope Protein in Brazil." *Revista Da Sociedade Brasileira de Medicina Tropical* 46 (1): 97–99. Accessed June 21, 2019. http://www.ncbi.nlm.nih.gov/pubmed/23563834.

Chen, Qiang. 2015. "Plant-Made Vaccines against West Nile Virus Are Potent, Safe, and Economically Feasible." *Biotechnology Journal* 10 (5): 671–80. https://doi.org/10.1002/biot.201400428.

Chu, J. J. H., R Rajamanonmani, J Li, R Bhuvanakantham, J Lescar, and M-L Ng. 2005. "Inhibition of West Nile Virus Entry by Using a Recombinant Domain III from the Envelope Glycoprotein." *Journal of General Virology* 86 (2): 405–12. https://doi.org/10.1099/vir.0.80411-0.

Chu, Jang-Hann J., Cern-Cher S. Chiang, and Mah-Lee Ng. 2007. "Immunization of Flavivirus West Nile Recombinant Envelope Domain

III Protein Induced Specific Immune Response and Protection against West Nile Virus Infection." *The Journal of Immunology* 178 (5): 2699–2705. https://doi.org/10.4049/jimmunol.178.5.2699.

Chua, Anthony JS, Cyrielle Vituret, Melvin LC Tan, Gaëlle Gonzalez, Pierre Boulanger, Mah-Lee Ng, and Saw-See Hong. 2013. "A Novel Platform for Virus-like Particle-Display of Flaviviral Envelope Domain III: Induction of Dengue and West Nile Virus Neutralizing Antibodies." *Virology Journal* 10 (1): 129. https://doi.org/10.1186/1743-422X-10-129.

Cielens, Indulis, Ludmila Jackevica, Arnis Strods, Andris Kazaks, Velta Ose, Janis Bogans, Paul Pumpens, and Regina Renhofa. 2014. "Mosaic RNA Phage VLPs Carrying Domain III of the West Nile Virus E Protein." *Molecular Biotechnology* 56 (5): 459–69. https://doi.org/10.1007/s12033-014-9743-3.

Coller BA, Pai V, Weeks-Levy C, Ogata S. 2012. Recombinant subunit West Nile virus vaccine for protections of human subjects. US20120141520, issued 2012. https://patentimages.storage.googleapis.com/41/84/ad/5e41003fd83aa5/AU2010257162B2.pdf.

Coutant, Frédéric, Marie-Pascale Frenkiel, Philippe Despres, and Pierre Charneau. 2008. "Protective Antiviral Immunity Conferred by a Nonintegrative Lentiviral Vector-Based Vaccine." Edited by Torbjorn Ramqvist. *PLoS ONE* 3 (12): e3973. https://doi.org/10.1371/journal.pone.0003973.

Dayan, Gustavo H., Joan Bevilacqua, Dorothy Coleman, Aileen Buldo, and George Risi. 2012. "Phase II, Dose Ranging Study of the Safety and Immunogenicity of Single Dose West Nile Vaccine in Healthy Adults ≥50 Years of Age." *Vaccine* 30 (47): 6656–64. https://doi.org/10.1016/j.vaccine.2012.08.063.

Dayan, Gustavo, Konstantin Pugachev, Joan Bevilacqua, Jean Lang, and Thomas Monath. 2013. "Preclinical and Clinical Development of a YFV 17 D-Based Chimeric Vaccine against West Nile Virus." *Viruses* 5 (12): 3048–70. https://doi.org/10.3390/v5123048.

Diamond, Michael S, Theodore C Pierson, and Daved H Fremont. 2008. "The Structural Immunology of Antibody Protection against West Nile

Virus." *Immunological Reviews* 225 (October): 212–25. https://doi.org/10.1111/j.1600-065X.2008.00676.x.

Durbin, Anna P., Peter F. Wright, Amber Cox, Wangeci Kagucia, Daniel Elwood, Susan Henderson, Kimberli Wanionek, Jim Speicher, Stephen S. Whitehead, and Alexander G. Pletnev. 2013. "The Live Attenuated Chimeric Vaccine RWN/DEN4Δ30 Is Well-Tolerated and Immunogenic in Healthy Flavivirus-Naïve Adult Volunteers." *Vaccine* 31 (48): 5772–77. https://doi.org/10.1016/j.vaccine.2013.07.064.

Filette, Marina De, Sebastian Ulbert, Mike Diamond, and Niek N Sanders. 2012. "Recent Progress in West Nile Virus Diagnosis and Vaccination." *Veterinary Research* 43 (1): 16. https://doi.org/10.1186/1297-9716-43-16.

Friedrich, Brian M., David W.C. Beasley, and Jai S. Rudra. 2016. "Supramolecular Peptide Hydrogel Adjuvanted Subunit Vaccine Elicits Protective Antibody Responses against West Nile Virus." *Vaccine* 34 (46): 5479–82. https://doi.org/10.1016/j.vaccine.2016.09.044.

Gershoni-Yahalom, Orly, Shimon Landes, Smadar Kleiman-Shoval, David Ben-Nathan, Michal Kam, Bat-El Lachmi, Yevgeny Khinich, et al. 2010. "Chimeric Vaccine Composed of Viral Peptide and Mammalian Heat-Shock Protein 60 Peptide Protects against West Nile Virus Challenge." *Immunology* 130 (4): 527–35. https://doi.org/10.1111/j.1365-2567.2010.03251.x.

He, Junyun, Li Peng, Huafang Lai, Jonathan Hurtado, Jake Stahnke, and Qiang Chen. 2014. "A Plant-Produced Antigen Elicits Potent Immune Responses against West Nile Virus in Mice." *BioMed Research International* 2014: 952865. https://doi.org/10.1155/2014/952865.

Iglesias, Maria Candela, Marie-Pascale Frenkiel, Karine Mollier, Philippe Souque, Philippe Despres, and Pierre Charneau. 2006. "A Single Immunization with a Minute Dose of a Lentiviral Vector-Based Vaccine Is Highly Effective at Eliciting Protective Humoral Immunity against West Nile Virus." *The Journal of Gene Medicine* 8 (3): 265–74. https://doi.org/10.1002/jgm.837.

Iyer, Arun V., Bapi Pahar, Marc J. Boudreaux, Nobuko Wakamatsu, Alma F. Roy, Vladimir N. Chouljenko, Abolghasem Baghian, Cristian

Apetrei, Preston A. Marx, and Konstantin G. Kousoulas. 2009. "Recombinant Vesicular Stomatitis Virus-Based West Nile Vaccine Elicits Strong Humoral and Cellular Immune Responses and Protects Mice against Lethal Challenge with the Virulent West Nile Virus Strain LSU-AR01." *Vaccine* 27 (6): 893–903. https://doi.org/10.1016/j.vaccine.2008.11.087.

Iyer, Arun V, and Konstantin G Kousoulas. 2013. "A Review of Vaccine Approaches for West Nile Virus." *International Journal of Environmental Research and Public Health* 10 (9): 4200–4223. https://doi.org/10.3390/ijerph10094200.

Kanai, R., K. Kar, K. Anthony, L. H. Gould, M. Ledizet, E. Fikrig, W. A. Marasco, R. A. Koski, and Y. Modis. 2006. "Crystal Structure of West Nile Virus Envelope Glycoprotein Reveals Viral Surface Epitopes." *Journal of Virology* 80 (22): 11000–8. https://doi.org/10.1128/JVI.01735-06.

Krol, Ewelina, Gabriela Brzuska, and Boguslaw Szewczyk. 2019. "Production and Biomedical Application of Flavivirus-like Particles." *Trends in Biotechnology* 0 (0). https://doi.org/10.1016/j.tibtech.2019.03.013.

Lai, Huafang, Amber M. Paul, Haiyan Sun, Junyun He, Ming Yang, Fengwei Bai, and Qiang Chen. 2018. "A Plant-Produced Vaccine Protects Mice against Lethal West Nile Virus Infection without Enhancing Zika or Dengue Virus Infectivity." *Vaccine* 36 (14): 1846–52. https://doi.org/10.1016/j.vaccine.2018.02.073.

Ledgerwood, Julie E, Theodore C Pierson, Sarah A Hubka, Niraj Desai, Steve Rucker, Ingelise J Gordon, Mary E Enama, et al. 2011. "A West Nile Virus DNA Vaccine Utilizing a Modified Promoter Induces Neutralizing Antibody in Younger and Older Healthy Adults in a Phase I Clinical Trial." *The Journal of Infectious Diseases* 203 (10): 1396–1404. https://doi.org/10.1093/infdis/jir054.

Ledizet, Michel, Kalipada Kar, Harald G. Foellmer, Tian Wang, Sandra L. Bushmich, John F. Anderson, Erol Fikrig, and Raymond A. Koski. 2005. "A Recombinant Envelope Protein Vaccine against West Nile

Virus." *Vaccine* 23 (30): 3915–24. https://linkinghub.elsevier.com/retrieve/pii/S0264410X05003518.

Lieberman, Michael M., David E. Clements, Steven Ogata, Gordon Wang, Gloria Corpuz, Teri Wong, Tim Martyak, et al. 2007. "Preparation and Immunogenic Properties of a Recombinant West Nile Subunit Vaccine." *Vaccine* 25 (3): 414–23. https://doi.org/10.1016/j.vaccine.2006.08.018.

Liu, Shiliang A., Muzammel Haque, Brent Stanfield, Frank M. Andrews, Alma A. Roy, and Konstantin G. Kousoulas. 2017. "A Recombinant Fusion Protein Consisting of West Nile Virus Envelope Domain III Fused In-Frame with Equine CD40 Ligand Induces Antiviral Immune Responses in Horses." *Veterinary Microbiology* 198 (January): 51–58. https://doi.org/10.1016/j.vetmic.2016.12.008.

Londono-Renteria, Berlin, and Tonya M. Colpitts. 2016. "A Brief Review of West Nile Virus Biology." In *Methods in Molecular Biology (Clifton, N.J.)*, 1435:1–13. https://doi.org/10.1007/978-1-4939-3670-0_1.

Magnusson, Sofia E., Karin H. Karlsson, Jenny M. Reimer, Silke Corbach-Söhle, Sameera Patel, Justin M. Richner, Norbert Nowotny, et al. 2014. "Matrix-M^{TM} Adjuvanted Envelope Protein Vaccine Protects against Lethal Lineage 1 and 2 West Nile Virus Infection in Mice." *Vaccine* 32 (7): 800–808. https://doi.org/10.1016/j.vaccine.2013.12.030.

Martín-Acebes, Miguel A, and Juan-Carlos Saiz. 2012. "West Nile Virus: A Re-Emerging Pathogen Revisited." *World Journal of Virology* 1 (2): 51–70. https://doi.org/10.5501/wjv.v1.i2.51.

Martin, Julie E, Theodore C Pierson, Sarah Hubka, Steve Rucker, Ingelise J Gordon, Mary E Enama, Charla A Andrews, et al. 2007. "A West Nile Virus DNA Vaccine Induces Neutralizing Antibody in Healthy Adults during a Phase 1 Clinical Trial." *The Journal of Infectious Diseases* 196 (12): 1732–40. https://doi.org/10.1086/523650.

Martina, Byron E., Penelopie Koraka, Petra van den Doel, Geert van Amerongen, Guus F. Rimmelzwaan, and Albert D.M.E. Osterhaus. 2008. "Immunization with West Nile Virus Envelope Domain III Protects Mice against Lethal Infection with Homologous and Heterologous Virus." *Vaccine* 26 (2): 153–57. http://www.ncbi.nlm.nih.gov/pubmed/18069096.

McDonald, William F., James W. Huleatt, Harald G. Foellmer, Duane Hewitt, Jie Tang, Priyanka Desai, Albert Price, et al. 2007. "A West Nile Virus Recombinant Protein Vaccine That Coactivates Innate and Adaptive Immunity." *The Journal of Infectious Diseases* 195 (11): 1607–17. https://doi.org/10.1086/517613.

Merino-Ramos, Teresa, Ana-Belén Blázquez, Estela Escribano-Romero, Rodrigo Cañas-Arranz, Francisco Sobrino, Juan-Carlos Saiz, and Miguel A Martín-Acebes. 2014. "Protection of a Single Dose West Nile Virus Recombinant Subviral Particle Vaccine against Lineage 1 or 2 Strains and Analysis of the Cross-Reactivity with Usutu Virus." *PloS One* 9 (9): e108056. https://doi.org/10.1371/journal.pone.0108056.

Nybakken, G. E., C. A. Nelson, B. R. Chen, M. S. Diamond, and D. H. Fremont. 2006. "Crystal Structure of the West Nile Virus Envelope Glycoprotein." *Journal of Virology* 80 (23): 11467–74. https://doi.org/10.1128/JVI.01125-06.

Ohtaki, Naohiro, Hidehiro Takahashi, Keiko Kaneko, Yasuyuki Gomi, Toyokazu Ishikawa, Yasushi Higashi, Takeshi Kurata, Tetsutaro Sata, and Asato Kojima. 2010. "Immunogenicity and Efficacy of Two Types of West Nile Virus-like Particles Different in Size and Maturation as a Second-Generation Vaccine Candidate." *Vaccine* 28 (40): 6588–96. https://doi.org/10.1016/J.VACCINE.2010.07.055.

Oliphant, T., G. E. Nybakken, S. K. Austin, Q. Xu, J. Bramson, M. Loeb, M. Throsby, D. H. Fremont, T. C. Pierson, and M. S. Diamond. 2007. "Induction of Epitope-Specific Neutralizing Antibodies against West Nile Virus." *Journal of Virology* 81 (21): 11828–39. https://doi.org/10.1128/JVI.00643-07.

Petersen, Lyle R, Aaron C Brault, and Roger S Nasci. 2013. "West Nile Virus: Review of the Literature." *JAMA* 310 (3): 308–15. https://doi.org/10.1001/jama.2013.8042.

Pierce, Kristen K., Stephen S. Whitehead, Beth D. Kirkpatrick, Palmtama L. Grier, Adrienne Jarvis, Heather Kenney, Marya P. Carmolli, et al. 2017. "A Live Attenuated Chimeric West Nile Virus Vaccine, RWN/DEN4Δ30, Is Well Tolerated and Immunogenic in Flavivirus-

Naive Older Adult Volunteers." *Journal of Infectious Diseases* 215 (1): 52–55. https://doi.org/10.1093/infdis/jiw501.

Pierson, Theodore C, Daved H Fremont, Richard J Kuhn, and Michael S Diamond. 2008. "Structural Insights into the Mechanisms of Antibody-Mediated Neutralization of Flavivirus Infection: Implications for Vaccine Development." *Cell Host & Microbe* 4 (3): 229–38. https://doi.org/10.1016/j.chom.2008.08.004.

Qiao, Ming, Mundrigi Ashok, Kristen A. Bernard, Gustavo Palacios, Z. Hong Zhou, W. Ian Lipkin, and T. Jake Liang. 2004. "Induction of Sterilizing Immunity against West Nile Virus (WNV), by Immunization with WNV-Like Particles Produced in Insect Cells." *The Journal of Infectious Diseases* 190 (12): 2104–8. https://doi.org/10.1086/425933.

Quintel, Benjamin K., Archana Thomas, Danae E. Poer DeRaad, Mark K. Slifka, and Ian J. Amanna. 2019. "Advanced Oxidation Technology for the Development of a Next-Generation Inactivated West Nile Virus Vaccine." *Vaccine* 37 (30): 4214–21. https://doi.org/10.1016/j.vaccine.2018.12.020.

Ramanathan, Mathura P., Michele A. Kutzler, Yuan-Chia Kuo, Jian Yan, Harrison Liu, Vidhi Shah, Amrit Bawa, et al. 2009. "Coimmunization with an Optimized IL15 Plasmid Adjuvant Enhances Humoral Immunity via Stimulating B Cells Induced by Genetically Engineered DNA Vaccines Expressing Consensus JEV and WNV E DIII." *Vaccine* 27 (32): 4370–80. https://doi.org/10.1016/j.vaccine.2009.01.137.

Rebollo, Belén, Teresa Pérez, Ana Camuñas, Elisa Pérez-Ramírez, Francisco Llorente, Maria Paz Sánchez-Seco, Miguel Ángel Jiménez-Clavero, and Ángel Venteo. 2018. "A Monoclonal Antibody to DIII E Protein Allowing the Differentiation of West Nile Virus from Other Flaviviruses by a Lateral Flow Assay." *Journal of Virological Methods* 260 (October): 41–44. https://doi.org/10.1016/j.jviromet.2018.06.016.

Scherwitzl, Iris, Juthathip Mongkolsapaja, and Gavin Screaton. 2017. "Recent Advances in Human Flavivirus Vaccines." *Current Opinion in Virology* 23 (April): 95–101. https://doi.org/10.1016/J.COVIRO.2017.04.002.

Sohrab, Sayed Sartaj, Mohd. Suhail, Mohammad A. Kamal, Azamal Husen, and Esam I. Azhar. 2017. "Recent Development and Future Prospects of Plant-Based Vaccines." *Current Drug Metabolism* 18 (July). https://doi.org/10.2174/1389200218666170711121810.

Spohn, Gunther, Gary T Jennings, Byron EE Martina, Iris Keller, Markus Beck, Paul Pumpens, Albert DME Osterhaus, and Martin F Bachmann. 2010. "A VLP-Based Vaccine Targeting Domain III of the West Nile Virus E Protein Protects from Lethal Infection in Mice." *Virology Journal* 7 (1): 146. https://doi.org/10.1186/1743-422X-7-146.

Tan, Lik Chern Melvin, Anthony Jin Shun Chua, Li Shan Liza Goh, Shu Min Pua, Yuen Kuen Cheong, and Mah Lee Ng. 2010. "Rapid Purification of Recombinant Dengue and West Nile Virus Envelope Domain III Proteins by Metal Affinity Membrane Chromatography." *Protein Expression and Purification* 74 (1): 129–37. https://doi.org/10.1016/j.pep.2010.06.015.

Taylor, Travis J., Fernando Diaz, Robert C. Colgrove, Kristen A. Bernard, Neal A. DeLuca, Sean P.J. Whelan, and David M. Knipe. 2016. "Production of Immunogenic West Nile Virus-like Particles Using a Herpes Simplex Virus 1 Recombinant Vector." *Virology* 496 (September): 186–93. https://doi.org/10.1016/J.VIROL.2016.06.006.

Tinker, Juliette, Jie Yan, Reece Knippel, Panos Panayiotou, and Kenneth Cornell. 2014. "Immunogenicity of a West Nile Virus DIII-Cholera Toxin A2/B Chimera after Intranasal Delivery." *Toxins* 6 (4): 1397–1418. https://doi.org/10.3390/toxins6041397.

Tripathi, Nagesh K., Divyanshi Karothia, Ambuj Shrivastava, Swati Banger, and Jyoti S. Kumar. 2018a. "Enhanced Production and Immunological Characterization of Recombinant West Nile Virus Envelope Domain III Protein." *New Biotechnology*. https://doi.org/10.1016/j.nbt.2018.05.002.

Tripathi, Nagesh K., and Ambuj Shrivastava. 2018b. "Recent Developments in Recombinant Protein–Based Dengue Vaccines." *Frontiers in Immunology* 9 (August): 1919. https://doi.org/10.3389/fimmu.2018.01919.

Tripathi, Nagesh K. 2016. "Production and Purification of Recombinant Proteins from Escherichia Coli." *ChemBioEng Reviews* 3 (3): 116–33. https://doi.org/10.1002/cben.201600002.

Ulbert, Sebastian. 2019. "West Nile Virus Vaccines – Current Situation and Future Directions." *Human Vaccines & Immunotherapeutics*, May, 21645515.2019.1621149. https://doi.org/10.1080/21645515.2019.1621149.

Ulbert, Sebastian, and Sofia E Magnusson. 2014. "Technologies for the Development of West Nile Virus Vaccines." *Future Microbiology* 9 (10): 1221–32. https://doi.org/10.2217/fmb.14.67.

Wang, T, J F Anderson, L A Magnarelli, S J Wong, R A Koski, and E Fikrig. 2001. "Immunization of Mice against West Nile Virus with Recombinant Envelope Protein." *Journal of Immunology (Baltimore, Md. : 1950)* 167 (9): 5273–77. https://doi.org/10.4049/jimmunol.167.9.5273.

Watts, Douglas M., Robert B. Tesh, Marina Siirin, Amelia Travassos da Rosa, Patrick C. Newman, David E. Clements, Steven Ogata, Beth-Ann Coller, Carolyn Weeks-Levy, and Michael M. Lieberman. 2007. "Efficacy and Durability of a Recombinant Subunit West Nile Vaccine Candidate in Protecting Hamsters from West Nile Encephalitis." *Vaccine* 25 (15): 2913–18. https://doi.org/10.1016/j.vaccine.2006.08.008.

Woods, Christopher W., Ana M. Sanchez, Geeta K. Swamy, Micah T. McClain, Lynn Harrington, Debra Freeman, Elizabeth A. Poore, et al. 2019. "An Observer Blinded, Randomized, Placebo-Controlled, Phase I Dose Escalation Trial to Evaluate the Safety and Immunogenicity of an Inactivated West Nile Virus Vaccine, HydroVax-001, in Healthy Adults." *Vaccine* 37 (30): 4222-4230. https://doi.org/10.1016/j.vaccine.2018.12.026.

Yap, Yun-Kiam, and Duncan R. Smith. 2010. "Strategies for the Plant-Based Expression of Dengue Subunit Vaccines." *Biotechnology and Applied Biochemistry* 57 (2): 47–53. https://doi.org/10.1042/BA20100248.

Zlatkovic, J., K. Stiasny, and F. X. Heinz. 2011. "Immunodominance and Functional Activities of Antibody Responses to Inactivated West Nile Virus and Recombinant Subunit Vaccines in Mice." *Journal of Virology* 85 (5): 1994–2003. https://doi.org/10.1128/JVI.01886-10.

In: West Nile Virus
Editor: Marinke van Verseveld

ISBN: 978-1-53616-589-0
© 2019 Nova Science Publishers, Inc.

Chapter 3

IMPACTS OF WEST NILE VIRUS ON THE YELLOW-BILLED MAGPIE AND OTHER BIRDS IN CALIFORNIA'S CENTRAL VALLEY

*Edward R. Pandolfino**
Sacramento, CA, US

ABSTRACT

Following the first major West Nile virus (WNV) outbreaks in the Central Valley of California (CV) in 2004-05, local populations of the Yellow-billed Magpie (*Pica nuttalli*) and several other bird species declined significantly. Magpie numbers declined to approximately one-half of their pre-WNV levels. Populations of several other birds, including the Loggerhead Shrike (*Lanius ludovicianus*), California Scrub-Jay (*Aphelocoma californica*), American Crow (*Corvus brachyrhynchos*), Oak Titmouse (*Baeolophus inornatus*), and House Finch (*Haemorhous mixicanus*), showed similar impacts. Most affected species showed signs

---

* Corresponding Author's E-mail: erpfromca@aol.com.

of recovery during the years following those outbreaks, however, Yellow-billed Magpie numbers have failed to recover to pre-WNV levels. Further, this magpie demonstrates persistent sensitivity to subsequent WNV outbreaks. These subsequent outbreaks have affected other species, but populations of those species appear to recover quickly following those outbreaks, while magpie numbers continue to decline. The range of the Yellow-billed Magpie is restricted to north-central California, and their range has constricted in recent decades with extirpation of some southern California populations. Therefore, the inability of this species to adapt to the presence of this virus is of significant conservation concern. In this chapter I review the impacts of WNV on several bird species and discuss the implications for the long-term survival the Yellow-billed Magpie.

Keywords: West Nile virus, birds, yellow-billed magpie

INTRODUCTION

As those of us on the west coast watched the inexorable spread of WNV eastward across North America following its first appearance in 1999 (Lanicotti et al. 1999, Anderson et al. 1999), concern grew about the potential impact of this virus on western birds. Many bird species are susceptible to WNV infection as shown both by surveys of wild birds (Komar et al. 2001, Reisen et al. 2004, Hayes et al. 2005, Nemeth et al. 2006, Engler et al. 2013) and experimental infection in laboratory settings (Komar et al. 2003, Bertelsen et al. 2004, Nemeth et al. 2006, Perez-Ramirez et al. 2013, de Oya et al. 2018). However, only a subset of bird families suffer high rates of mortality from these infections (McLean 2006, LaDeau et al. 2007, George et al. 2015). These sensitive families include finchs (family Fringillidae; Komar et al. 2003, George et al. 2015), raptors (families Accipitridae and Strigidae: hawks and owls; Fitzgerald et al. 2003, Saito et al. 2010, Dusek et al. 2010), and titmice (family Paridae: includes chickadees; La Deau et al. 2007, Airola et al. 2007, George et al. 2015). However, corvids (family Corvidae: crows, jays, magpies, etc.), demonstrate the highest levels of infection and mortality (Komar et al. 2003, Bonter and Hochachka 2003, Yaremych et al. 2004, LaDeau et al. 2007).

The spread of WNV across the continent has been associated with declines in populations of many bird species (McLean 2006, George et al. 2015), with the American Crow and other corvids demonstrating the most significant declines (Bonter and Hochachka 2003, Caffrey 2003, Caffrey et al. 2005, McLean 2006). Of the western members of this family, the Yellow-billed Magpie has the second most restricted range, being endemic to California and mainly limited to the Sacramento and San Joaquin valleys and the central Coast Range (Koenig and Reynolds 2009). In recent decades, this species' range has constricted further (Roberson 1985, Lehman 1994, Koenig and Reynolds 2009, Crosbie et al. 2014) with the extirpation of some southern California populations (Garrett and Dunn 1981, Lehman 1994).

WNV was first documented in California in 2003 (Reisen et al. 2004), but it was not until the summers of 2004 and 2005 that it reached epidemic levels in the state (CDPH 2019). The typically very warm CV experienced some of the highest levels of human and bird infections of any region in the state (Foss et al. 2015, CDPH 2019). In this chapter I review the evidence for impacts of WNV on bird populations in the CV, with particular emphasis on the endemic Yellow-billed Magpie.

METHODS

Study Area

The Central Valley, lying between the Sierra Nevada to the west and the Coast Ranges to the east, is the largest geographic feature in California, approximately 600 km long and 60km wide (Figure 1). It consists of two large river valleys (the Sacramento and San Joaquin valleys) and the Sacramento–San Joaquin River Delta, where these two river systems merge and flow into the San Francisco Bay estuary. Winters in the CV are generally wet and mild and summers are hot and dry. Winter tempeatures rarely drop below freezing and most of the annual rainfall occurs between November and March. Dominant land cover consists of (percentages approximate):

- grassland/oak savanna, mostly around the valley edges (35%);
- intense forms of agriculture (orchards, vineyards, row crops; 25%);
- less intense agriculture (hay, winter wheat, irrigated pasture; 15%);
- rice (10%);
- developed (urban, suburban, rural residential; 10%)
- managed wetland (3%).

Land cover types increasing at the highest rates in recent decades are orchards, vineyards, and developed, mostly at the expense of grassland/savanna habitats (Cameron et al. 2014).

Data Sources

Much of the data on bird populations cited in this chapter came from 17 Christmas Bird Counts (CBC; NAS 2010) located in the CV (Figure 1). These Count Circles have been run consistently over the past four decades. Other data sources used include the Breeding Bird Survey (BBS; Sauer et al. 2017) and the California Department of Public Health (CDPH 2019; for human infection cases, dead birds, and prevalence of WNV among mosquitos).

WNV IMPACTS ON BIRDS

Initial Impacts

The first appearance of WNV in California in 2003 (Reisen et al. 2004) was associated with only a small number of reports of human infections or WNV-positive dead birds (3 and 96, respectively; CDPH 2019).

Impacts of West Nile Virus on the Yellow-Billed Magpie ... 97

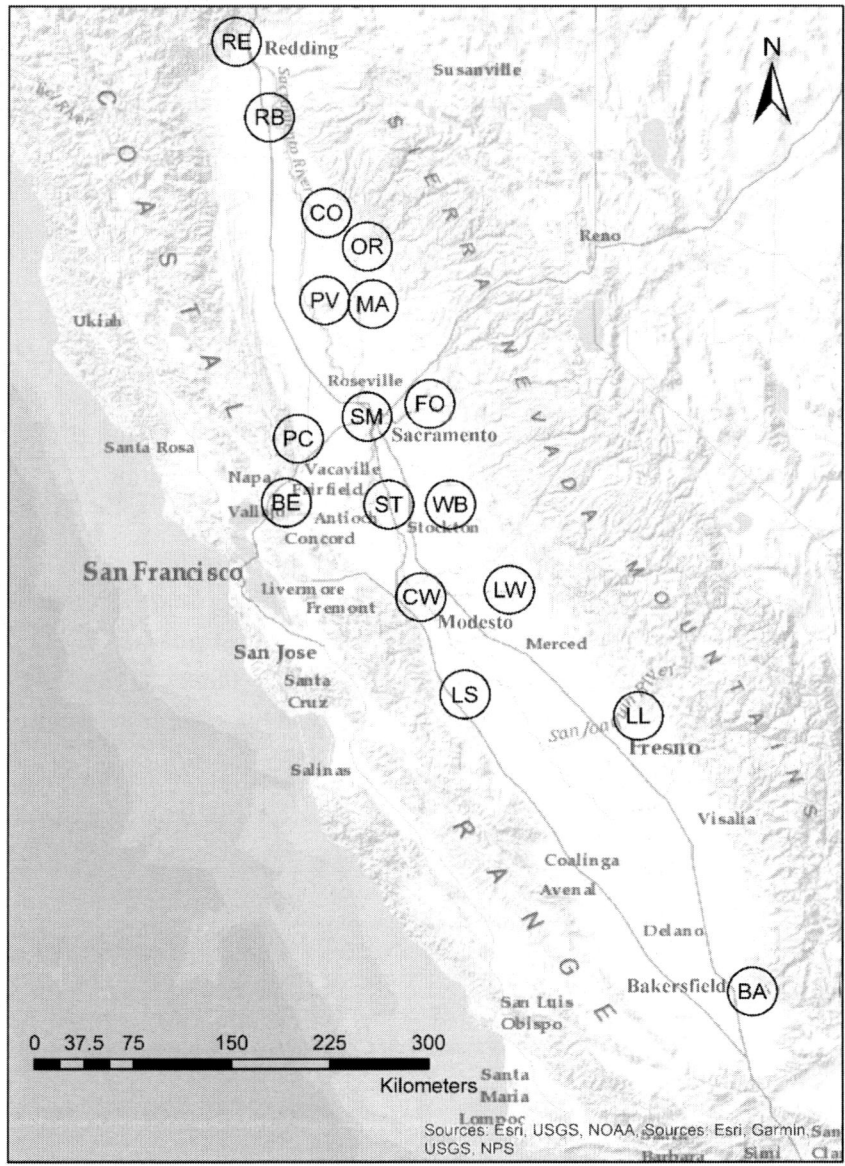

Figure 1. The Central Valley of California showing locations of 17 Christmas Bird Count circles within the valley. Count Circles north to south are: RE = Redding; RB = Red Bluff; CO = Chico; OR = Oroville; PV = Peace Valley; MA = Marysville; FO = Folsom; SM = Sacramento; PC = Putah Creek; BE = Benicia; ST = Stockton; WB = Wallace-Bellota; CW = Caswell-Westley; LW = LaGrange-Waterford; LS = Los Banos; LL = Lost Lake; BA = Bakersfield.

However, the virus spread quickly and reached outbreak levels in the summers of 2004 and 2005. Cases of human infections statewide reached 779 in 2004 and 880 in 2005 and the number of dead birds infected with the virus exceeded 3000 in each of those years (CDPH 2019). In the CV, the virus was less common than statewide in 2004 (39 human cases), but reached high levels in 2005 (492 human cases; CDPH 2019).

By 2005 anecdotal reports began to appear on various birding listserves citing few Yellow-billed Magpies in locations where they were typically common, and dramatically low numbers from CBCs. Table 1 compares the average number of magpies recorded on CV CBCs for the 20 years before the 2005 WNV outbreak to the numbers recorded during the winter of 2005-06. However, it was not until 2007 that the first documentation of declines in bird populations was published (Airola et al. 2007, Koenig et al. 2007).

Table 1. Comparison of the number of Yellow-billed Magpies recorded on CV CBCs for the 20-year period prior to the summer of 2005 to the number recorded during the winter 2005 - 06 count (includes only count circles within the normal Yellow-billed Magpie range)

	20-year Ave.	Wtr 05-06
Redding	98	38
Red Bluff	219	30
Chico	519	153
Oroville	48	8
Peace Valley	173	79
Marysville	270	179
Folsom	184	67
Sacramento	1231	406
Putah Creek	571	332
Wallace-Bellota	254	184
Stockton	192	137
Caswell-Westley	1351	385
La Grange-Waterford	304	142
Los Banos	500	183

Airola et al. (2007) used CBC data from the lower Sacramento Valley (nothern portions of the CV) to document declines of 38-48% for the California Scrub-Jay, Yellow-billed Magpie, American Crow, and Oak Titmouse, all members of families known to be susceptible to WNV. They also looked at results for nine species from families thought to be resistant to the virus and found that one species (Califonia Quail; *Callipepla californica*) had increased significantly, two declined significantly (Bushtit; *Psaltriparus minimus* and White-breasted Nuthatch; *Sitta carolinensis*), while six others showed non-significant changes. Koenig et al. (2007) used data from BBS routes in California to demonstrate widespread declines in many WNV-sensitive species, with four corvid species (Steller's Jay; *Cyanocitta stelleri*, California Scrub-Jay, Yellow-billed Magpie, and American Crow) showing particularly large declines.

Work by Crosbie et al. (2008) focused on the Yellow-billed Magpie and showed declines of 22% based on BBS data and 42% using CBC data. They also collected data from several known roosting sites, all of which showed reduced numbers of magpies. They tested 21 living Yellow-billed Magpies in 2006 and found only one had neutralizing antibodies against WNV.

CBC data from 17 CV CBC circles for the three winters following the 2005 summer WNV outbreak provided further evidence of declines in California Scrub-Jays, Yellow-billed Magpies, and American Crows, as well as Loggerhead Shrikes (Pandolfino 2008a). Yellow-billed Magpies showed the largest decline (50%).

A second study (Pandolfino 2008b) focused on the Loggerhead Shrike in the CV and confirmed declines using both CBC and BBS data, with the counties having the highest rates of WNV showing the largest shrike declines.

Wheeler et al. (2009) looked at correlations between bird carcass counts, seropositivity, and BBS population trends in California and determined that five species (Black-crowned Night-Heron; *Nycticorax nycticorax*, California Scrub-Jay, Yellow-billed Magpie, American Crow, and House Finch) were at highest risk for impacts from ongoing WNV activity in the state.

Table 2. Changes in abundance of the Yellow-billed Magpie during the years immediately following the first outbreaks of WNV in California

Data Source	Location	Change	Citation
CBC	CV	-48%	Airola et al. 2007
BBS	Statewide	-34%[1]	Koenig et al. 2007
CBC	CV/Coast Range	-48%	Crosbie et al. 2008
BBS	CV/Coast Range	-22%	Crosbie et al. 2008
CBC	CV	-48% to -68%	Pandolfino 2008a, 2009, 2010
Road Surveys	CV	-83%	Smallwood & Nakamoto 2009
BBS	CV	-70%[2]	Wheeler et al. 2009

[1]Percent decline from W. Koenig, pers. comm. Citation reported as log-transformed value.
[2]Approximate value based on visual examination of published trend curve.

Smallwood and Nakamoto (2009) compared results from roadside surveys conducted in the Sacramento Valley in the early 1990s to those after 2004 and found declines of 83% in the Yellow-billed Magpie, 63% for the American Crow, and 63% for the Loggerhead Shrike.

Regardless of the sources of data or the geographic coverage, these studies all noted significant declines in the abundance of Yellow-billed Magpies immediately following the appearance of WNV in California (Table 2).

Recovery?

Continued monitoring of results from CV CBCs (Pandolfino 2009 and 2010) provided evidence that the populations of the Oak Titmouse, American Crow, and California Scrub-Jay were recovering to levels at or above their pre-WNV averages. In contrast, Yellow-billed Magpie and Loggerhead Shrike numbers showed no signs of recovery, both remaining at approximately half their pre-WNV levels (Figure 2). To examine this further, I used both CBC and BBS data for the CV to look at Yellow-billed Magpie populations through 2012 (Pandolfino 2013). Both sources confirmed the lack of any sign of recovery of magpie numbers in the CV (Figure 3). The post-WNV declines were widespread with all 17 CBC circles showing declines ranging from 39-96% and all 10 BBS routes showing declines of 30-87% following the 2005 outbreak. It is more difficult to draw conclusions about recovery of the Loggerhead Shrike due to a history of declines that pre-date the arrival of WNV.

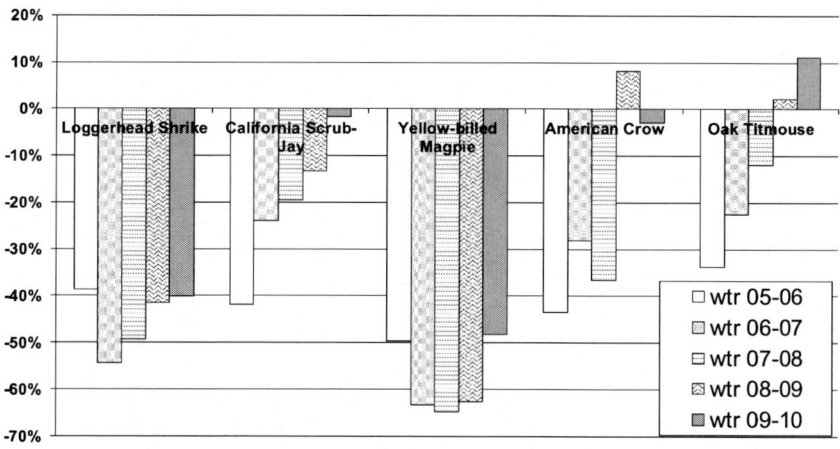

Figure 2. Comparison of the pre-WNV abundances (10-year average) to the abundances for the five winters following the 2005 outbreak for five species (based on birds/party hour from 17 Central Valley CBC circles) (Reprinted from Pandolfino 2010 by permission from Central Valley Bird Club Bulletin).

WNV continues to be present in our area and virus activity has periodically spiked since the initial 2004-05 outbreaks (Foss et al. 2015, CDPH 2019). Data from human infection reports, WNV-positive dead birds, and virus-positive mosquitos suggest peaks in 2007, 08, 12, 14, and 16 in the CV or statewide (Foss et al. 2015, CDPH 2019, Pandolfino 2018). Data from bird banding stations across North America showed that, while many species were impacted by WNV, they could generally be grouped into those whose numbers recovered after initial exposure and those showing persistent impacts on the population (George et al. 2015).

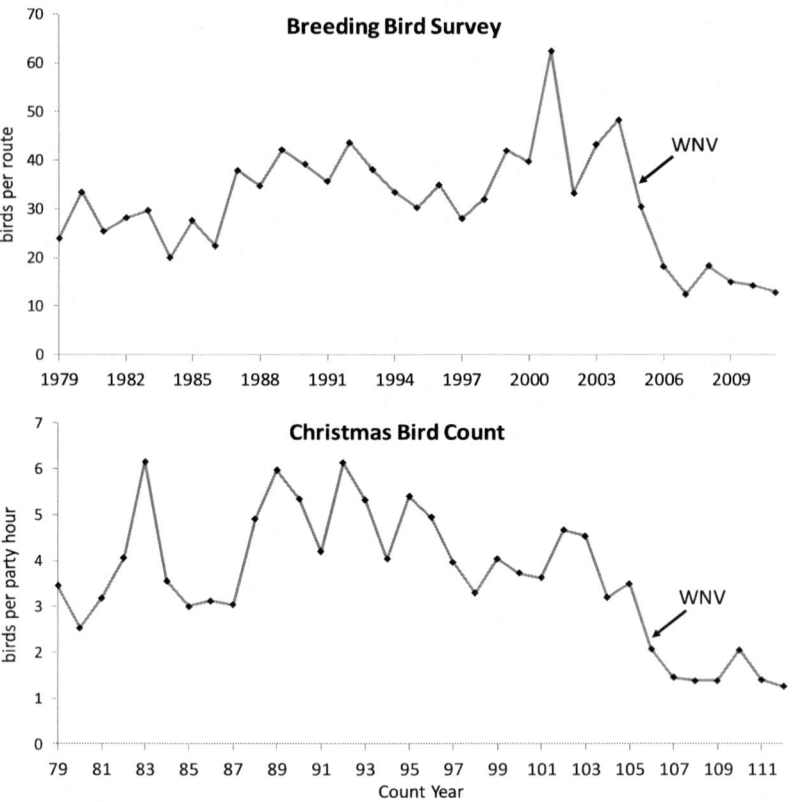

Figure 3. Trends in abundance of the Yellow-billed Magpie in California's Central Valley before and after the appearance of West Nile virus (Reprinted from Pandolfino 2013 by permission from Western Birds).

With magpie populations showing no signs of recovery, this raises the possiblity that this species continues to be susceptible to further declines as WNV activity waxes and wanes. To examine this, I looked for correlations between changes magpie abundance in the CV and WNV activity from 2000 - 2016. I found that the three corvid species (Califonia Scrub-Jay, Yellow-billed Magpie, and American Crow) each showed a significant negative correlation between virus activity (measured by human cases reported in the

CV) and abundance from CBCs conducted the following winter (Pandolfino 2018). However, it appeared that the numbers of jays and crows rebounded in years following the spike in virus activity, while magpie numbers did not. Data on ten other species considered to be relatively resistant to WNV showed no correlation with virus activity. The Oak Titmouse, a WNV-sensitive species, showed a negative correlation that approached, but did not reach significance ($p = 0.07$).

Implications for the Future

A substantial and growing body of evidence suggests that the California endemic Yellow-billed Magpie is at continuing risk of further declines, and perhaps even of extinction. Examination of WNV-infected dead magpies indicates a very rapid onset of morbidity and mortality, with many different organ systems affected (Ernest et al. 2010). This finding is consistent with those from experimentally infected Black-billed Magpies (*Pica hudsonia*; Komar et al. 2003, de Oya et al. 2018), a closely-related species.

Even some years after the intial appearance of WNV in the state, every study finds that the prevalance of WNV in dead Yellow-billed Magpies is the highest of any species tested (Crosbie et al. 2008, Wheeler et al. 2009, Ernest et al. 2010, Foss et al. 2015). Of most concern, almost no living magpies appear to have developed immunity to the virus (Crosbie et al. 2008, Ernest et al. 2010). Population studies show recovery of most other species (Pandolfino 2008 and 2010, George et al. 2015) and suggest that a WNV-resistant population of some (including some corvids) has emerged (Pandolfino 2018). It seems that, either nearly all infected Yellow-billed Magpies are dying, or that they are largely incapable of mounting an immune response to the virus. Without a reservoir of virus-resistant magpies, the ongoing presence of WNV is likely to produce additional population declines. Ernest et al. (2010) suggested that "Yellow-billed Magpies may be at risk of a population decline and bottleneck event".

Two other factors, their very restricted range and generally sedentary nature (Koenig and Reynolds 2009), put this species at particular risk. Historically, most avian extinctions have been based on a combination of effects, rather than a single factor (Fuller 2001). Even prior to the appearance of WNV in the state, the range of this bird was constricting, mainly attributed to habitat conversion (Lehman 1994, Koenig and Reynolds 2009, Crosbie et al. 2014). However, CBC data from the CV showed that population was generally stable prior to WNV (Pandolfino 2008a, Pandolfino and Handel 2018). Indeed, while sizable portions of their natural oak savanna habitat are being converted to other, incompatible uses (Cameron et al. 2014), this species has adapted well to habitats such as golf courses and parks. Assuming that, ultimately, a population of WNV-resistant Yellow-billed Magpies emerges, the species may persist, even if at a fraction of their former population levels.

REFERENCES

Airola, D. A., S. Hampton and T. Manolis. 2007. Effects of West Nile virus on sensitive species in the lower Sacramento Valley, California: An evaluation using Christmas Bird Counts. *Central Valley Bird Club Bulletin,* 10:1 - 22.

Anderson, J. F., T. G. Andreadis, C. R. Vossbrinck, S. Tirrell, E. M. Wakem and R. A. French. 1999. Isolation of West Nile virus from mosquitoes, crows, and a Cooper's Hawk in Connecticut. *Science,* 286:2331 - 2333.

Bertelsen, M. F., R.-A. Olberg, G. J. Crawshaw, A. Dibernardo, L. R. Linsay, M. Drebot and I. K. Barker. 2004. West Nile viruse infection in the eastern Loggerhead Shrike (*Lanius ludovicianus migrans*): Pathology, epidemiology, and immunization. *Journal of Wildlife Diseases,* 40:538 - 542.

Bonter, D. N. and W. M. Hochachka. 2003. Combined data of Project Feederwatch and Christmas Bird Count indicate declines of chickadees and corvids: possible impacts of West Nile virus. *American Birds,* (103rd Christmas Bird Count 2002-2003):22 - 25.

Caffrey, C. 2003. Determining impacts of West Nile virus on crows and other birds. *American Birds,* (l03rd Christmas Bird Count 2002-2003):12 - 13.

Caffrey, C. S., C. R. Smith and T. J. Weston. 2005. West Nile virus devastates an American Crow population. *Condor,* 107:128 - 132.

California Department of Public Health (CDPH). 2019. *California West Nile virus webiste.* http://westnile.ca.gov/.

Cameron, D. R., J. Marty and R. F. Holland. 2014. Whither the rangeland?: Protection and conversion in California's rangeland ecosystems. *PLoS One,* 9(8): e103468; doi 10.1371/ journal.pone.0103468.

Centers for Disease Control (CDC). 2012. *West Nile Virus: Statistics, surveillance, and control archive,* http://www.cdc.gov/ncidod/dvbid/westnile/surv&control.htm [accessed Jan 2013].

Crosbie, S. P., W. D. Koenig, W. Reisen, V. L. Kramer, L. Marcus, R. Carney, E. R. Pandolfino, G. M. Bolen, L. R. Crosbie, D. A. Bell and H. B. Ernest. 2008. A preliminary assessment: Impact of West Nile virus on the Yellow-billed Magpie, a California endemic. *Auk,* 125: 542 - 550.

Crosbie, S. P., L. E. Souza, H. B. Ernest. 2014. Abundance and distribution of the Yellow-billed Magpie. *Western Birds,* 45:100 - 111.

de Oya, N. J., M.-C. Camacho, A.-B. Blazquez, J. Francisco L.-B., J.-C. Saiz, U. Hofle and E. Escribano-Romero. 2018. High susceptibility of magpie (*Pica pica*) to experimental infection with lineage 1 and 2 West Nile virus. *PLoS Neglected Tropical Diseases,* 12: https://doi.org/10.1371/journal.pntd.0006394.

Dusek, R. J., W. M. Iko, E. K. Hofmeister. 2010. Occurrence of West Nile virus infection in raptors at the Salton Sea, California. *Journal of Wildlife Diseases,* 46:889 - 895.

Engler, O., G. Savini, A. Papa, J. Figuerola, M. H. Groschup, H. Kampen, J. Medlock, A. Vaux, A. J. Wilson, D. Werner. 2013. European surveillance for West Nile virus in mosquito populations. *International Journal of Enviromental Research and Public Health,* 10:4869 - 4895.

Ernest, H. B., L. W. Woods and B. R. Hoar. 2010. Pathology associated with West Nile virus infections in the Yellow-billed Magpie (*Pica nuttalli*): A California endemic bird. *Journal of Wildlife Diseases,* 46:401 - 408.

Fitzgerald, S. D., J. S. Patterson, M. Kiupel, H. A. Simmons, S. D. Grimes, C. F. Sarver, R. M. Fulton, B. A. Steficek, T. M. Cooley, J. P. Massey and J. G. Sikarskie. 2003. Clinical and pathological features of West Nile virus infection in native North American owls (Family Strigidae). *Avian Disease,* 47:602 - 610.

Foss, L. K. Padgett, W. K. Reisen, A. Kjemtrup, J. Ogawa and V. Kramer. 2015. West Nile virus-related trends in avian mortality in California, USA, 2003-12. *Journal of Wildlife Diseases,* 51:576 - 588. doi: 10.7589/2014-06-144.

Fuller, E. 2001. *Extinct Birds.* Cornell University Press, Ithaca, NY.

Garrett, K. G. and J. Dunn. 1981. Birds of Southern California: Status and Distribution. Los Angeles Audubon Society, Los Angeles, CA.

George, T. L., R. J. Harrigan, J. A. LaManna, D. F. DeSante, J. F. Saracco and T. B. Smith. 2015. Persistent impacts of West Nile virus on North American bird populations. *Proceedings National Academy of Science,* 112:14290 - 14294. www.pnas.org/cgi/doi/10.1073/pnas.1507747112.

Hayes, E. B., N. Komar, R. S. Nasci, S. P. Montgomery, D. R. O'Leary, G. L. Campbell. 2005. Epidemiology and transmission dynamics of West Nile virus disease. *Emerging Infectious Diseases,* 11:1167 - 1173.

Koenig, W. D., L. Marcus, T. W. Scott and J. L. Dickinson. 2007. West Nile virus and California breeding bird declines. *EcoHealth,* 4:18 - 24.

Koenig, W. D. and M. D. Reynolds. 2009. Yellow-billed Magpie (Pica nuttalli), version 2.0. In *The Birds of North America,* (A. F. Poole, Editor). Cornell Lab of Ornithology, Ithaca, NY, USA. https://doi.org/10.2173/bna.180.

Komar, N., J. Burns, C. Dean, N. A. Panella, S. Dusza and B. Cherry. 2001. Serologic evidence for West Nile virus infection in birds in Staten Island, New York, after an outbreak in 2000. *Vector-Borne and Zoonotic Diseases,* 1:191 - 196.

Komar, N. S. Langevin, S. Hinten, N. M. Nemeth, E. Edwards, D. L. Hettler, B. S. Davis, R. A. Bowen and M. L. Bunning. 2003. Experimental infection of North American birds with the New York 1999 strain of West Nile virus. *Emerging Infectious Diseases,* 9:311 - 322.

LaDeau, S. L., A. M. Kilpatrick, P. P. Marra. 2007. West Nile virus emergence and large-scale declines of North American bird populations. *Nature,* 447:710 - 713.

Lanciotti, R. S., J. T. Roehrig, V. Deubel, J. Smith, M. Parker and K. Steele. 1999. Origin of the West Nile virus responsible for an outbreak of encephalitis in the northeastern United States. *Science,* 286:2333 - 2337.

Lehman, P. E. 1994. The Birds of Santa Barbara County, California. Vertebrate Museum, University of California, Santa Barbara, CA.

McLean, R. G. 2006. West Nile virus in North American birds. *Ornithological Monographs,* 60:44 - 64.

National Audubon Society (NAS). 2010. *The Christmas Bird Count historical results;* netapp.audubon.org/cbcobservation/.

Nemeth, N., D. Gould, R. Bowen and N. Komar. 2006. Natural and experimental West Nile virus infection in five raptor species. *Journal of Wildlife Diseases,* 42:1 - 13. https://doi.org/10.7589/0090-3558-42.1.1

Pandolfino, E. R. 2008a. Review of the 108th Christmas Bird Count in the Central Valley of California: December 2007-January 2008. *Central Valley Bird Club Bulletin,* 11:53 - 61.

Pandolfino, E. R. 2008b. Population trends of the Loggerhead Shrike in California: Possible impact of West Nile virus in the Central Valley. *Central Valley Bird Club Bulletin,* 11:37 - 44.

Pandolfino, E. R. 2009. Review of the 109th Christmas Bird Count in the Central Valley of California: December 2008-January 2009. *Central Valley Bird Club Bulletin,* 12:53 - 62.

Pandolfino, E. R. 2010. Review of the 110th Christmas Bird Count in the Central Valley of California: December 2009-January 2010. *Central Valley Bird Club Bulletin,* 13:25 - 34.

Pandolfino, E. R. 2013. Lack of recovery of the Yellow-billed Magpie from the West Nile virus in California's Central Valley. *Western Birds,* 44:143 - 147.

Pandolfino, E. R. 2018. Continuing impacts of West Nile virus on birds of California's Central Valley. *Central Valley Bird Club Bulletin,* 20:101 - 109.

Pandolfino, E. R. and C. M. Handel. 2018. Population trends of birds wintering in the Central Valley of California, in *Trends and traditions: Avifaunal change in western North America,* (W. D. Shuford, R. E. Gill Jr., and C. M. Handel, eds.), pp. 215-235. *Studies of Western Birds,* 3. Western Field Ornithologists, Camarillo, CA.

Perez-Ramirez, E., F. Llorente and M. A. Jimenez-Clavero. 2014. Experimental infections of wild birds with West Nile virus. *Viruses,* 6:752 - 781. doi:10.3390/v6020752.

Reisen, W. H., R. Lothrop, M. Chiles, C. Madon, L. Cossen, S. Woods, S. Husted, V. Kramer and J. Edman. 2004. West Nile virus in California. *Emerging Infectious Diseases,* (online serial). www.cdc.gov/ncidod/EID/voIIOn08/04-0077.htm.

Roberson, D. 1985. Monterey Birds. Monterey Peninsula Audubon Society, Carmel, CA.

Saito, E. K., L. Sileo, D. E. Green, C. U. Meteyer, G. S. McLaughlin, K. A. Converse, D. E. Docherty. 2007. Raptor mortality due to West Nile virus in the United States, 2002. *Journal of Wildlife Diseases,* 43: 206 - 213.

Sauer, J. R., Niven, D. K., Hines, J. E., Ziolkowski, D. J., Jr., Pardieck, K. L., Fallon, J. E. and Link, W. A. 2017. *The North American Breeding Bird Survey, results and analysis,* 1966 - 2015, version 2.07.2017. USGS Patuxent Wildl. Res. Ctr., Laurel, MD. www.mbr-pwrc.usgs.gov/bbs/trend/tf15.html.

Smallwood, K. S. and B. Nakamoto. 2009. Impacts of the West Nile virus epizootic on the Yellow-billed Magpie, American Crow, and other birds in the Sacramento Valley, California. 2009. *Condor,* 111:247 - 254.

Wheeler, S. S., C. M. Barker, Y. Fang, M. V. Armijos, B. D. Carroll, S. Husted, W. O. Johnson and W. K. Reisen. 2009. Differential impact of West Nile virus on California birds. *Condor,* 111:1 - 20.

Yaremych, S. A., R. E. Warner, P. C. Mankin, J. D. Brawn, A. Raim and R. Novak. 2004. West Nile virus and high death rate in American Crows. *Emerging Infectious Diseases,* (online serial) http://www .cdc.gov /ncidodlElD/voll Ono4/03-0499 .htm.

INDEX

A

agent-based model, v, vii, 1, 2, 3, 17, 29, 31, 33, 34
algorithm, 6, 15, 29, 53
American crow, ix, 4, 51, 93, 95, 99, 100, 102, 105, 108
amplitude, 27, 52
antibody, viii, 68, 71, 73, 76, 77, 79, 80
antigen, 71, 73, 74, 75, 78, 79
antiviral drugs, viii, 67
Aphelocoma californica, ix, 93
authorities, 28, 29
avian, viii, 2, 13, 24, 104, 106

B

bacteria, viii, 67, 79
Baeolophus inornatus, ix, 93
birds, v, vii, ix, 2, 3, 4, 5, 6, 8, 10, 11, 12, 13, 14, 16, 17, 21, 24, 28, 29, 30, 35, 40, 41, 44, 45, 46, 48, 49, 50, 51, 61, 65, 93, 94, 96, 98, 101, 102, 104, 105, 106, 107, 108
bloodstream, 48, 49
breeding, 13, 26, 30, 40, 59, 106
breeding bird survey, 96, 108
Bushtit, 99

C

calibration, 5, 11, 14, 15, 16, 29, 52, 53, 54
Califonia quail, 99
California, v, ix, 36, 39, 62, 64, 65, 66, 93, 95, 96, 97, 99, 100, 102, 103, 104, 105, 106, 107, 108
California scrub-jay, ix, 93, 99, 100
Callipepla californica, 99
candidates, viii, 67, 68, 72, 74, 75, 77, 80
carbon dioxide, 6, 14, 18
cell culture, 71, 78, 80
cellular difference equation, v, vii, 1, 2, 5, 27
Central Valley, v, ix, 93, 95, 97, 101, 102, 104, 107, 108
Christmas bird counts, 96, 104
chromatography, 70, 79
classes, 11, 42, 43
climate, 23, 28
clinical trials, 72, 74, 80

color, iv, 24, 55
communities, viii, 2, 15, 16, 28, 52
community, 3, 4, 15, 40, 52
complexity, 5, 13, 45
conservation, ix, 94
Corvidae, 94
corvids, 49, 94, 95, 103, 104
Corvus brachyrhynchos, ix, 93
cost, 28, 69, 81
Cyanocitta stelleri, 99

D

death rate, 27, 49, 51, 108
dengue, 29, 72
depth, 26, 80
differential equations, 4, 5, 28
diseases, 26, 29
distribution, viii, 2, 20, 21, 23, 46, 105
DNA, 68, 71, 73, 74, 76, 77, 78, 80, 85, 86, 88
Drosophila, 70, 73, 74
drought, 27, 29

E

encephalitis, viii, 67, 107
endemic, 95, 103, 105
envelope domain III, v, vii, ix, 67, 68, 77, 78, 80, 83, 86, 89
envelope protein, 81, 82, 85, 86, 90
environment, viii, 2, 4, 29, 30, 59
epidemiology, 4, 13, 17, 104
epitopes, viii, 68, 69, 75, 76
Escherichia coli (E. coli), 68, 69, 72, 73, 77, 78
evidence, 95, 99, 100, 103, 106

F

families, 49, 94, 99
fitness, 15, 16, 53, 54
food, 13, 14, 40
fusion, 69, 73, 78, 81

H

habitat, 3, 10, 11, 16, 26, 31, 40, 54, 56, 60, 96, 104
Haemorhous mixicanus, ix, 93
health, 4, 29, 32, 64
horses, 74, 79
host, vii, viii, 3, 10, 11, 12, 13, 14, 18, 31, 37, 40, 42, 44, 45, 62, 67, 69, 70, 80
House, ix, 35, 36, 51, 93, 99
house finch, ix, 35, 51, 93, 99
human, viii, 2, 3, 4, 5, 8, 9, 11, 18, 28, 29, 53, 54, 55, 67, 68, 71, 72, 73, 80, 83, 95, 96, 98, 101, 102
humoral immunity, 74, 79

I

immune response, 35, 73, 76, 77, 78, 80, 83, 84, 85, 86, 103
immunity, viii, 38, 63, 68, 74, 75, 79, 80, 83, 84, 87, 88, 103
immunization, 79, 80, 104
immunogen, 69, 79
immunogenicity, 73, 74, 78
incubation period, 27, 56
individuals, 4, 73
induction, 69, 70, 73, 77, 79
infections, 2, 10, 12, 13, 16, 17, 21, 24, 25, 26, 27, 29, 40, 44, 45, 46, 47, 48, 49, 50, 51, 71, 73, 74, 77, 78, 80, 94, 95, 96, 98, 101, 104, 105, 106, 107, 108
insect cell, viii, 67, 68, 69, 73, 74, 75, 76, 88

L

landscape, 6, 8, 10, 11, 16, 28, 40, 54, 56, 59
Lanius ludovicianus, ix, 93, 104
larvae, 10, 19, 26, 41, 78, 79
loggerhead shrike, ix, 93, 99, 100, 101, 104, 107

M

magnitude, 40, 73
mammals, 40, 41
mice, 73, 74, 75, 76, 77, 78, 79, 80
migration, vii, 2, 6, 8, 10, 11, 18, 28, 29, 40
modelling, viii, 2, 3, 4, 13, 17, 27, 56
models, vii, viii, 2, 3, 4, 5, 13, 17, 41, 56, 73
modifications, 5, 29
morbidity, 103
mortality, 2, 35, 49, 94, 103, 106, 108
mosquitoes, viii, 2, 3, 4, 10, 11, 12, 14, 15, 16, 17, 18, 19, 20, 21, 22, 23, 24, 26, 27, 29, 30, 31, 40, 41, 42, 44, 45, 48, 52, 53, 54, 56, 59, 96, 101, 104

N

Nycticorax nycticorax, 99

O

oak savanna, 96, 104
oak titmouse, ix, 93, 99, 100, 103
optimization, 15, 53, 54, 70

P

peptide, 69, 76, 79
permission, iv, 101, 102
Pica hudsonia, 103
plants, viii, 67, 68, 69, 80
policymakers, viii, 2
pools, 29, 52
population, viii, 2, 3, 4, 6, 8, 10, 11, 12, 13, 15, 16, 17, 18, 21, 24, 26, 28, 29, 31, 40, 53, 55, 57, 99, 102, 103, 104, 105
precipitation, 26, 27
prevalance, 103
prevention, vii, 2
probability, 8, 10, 11, 12, 13, 24, 30, 41, 44, 45, 46, 47, 48, 50, 51
propagation, 5, 18, 21, 24, 29
protection, 73, 74, 76, 77, 78, 80
protein expression, 70
proteins, viii, 67, 68, 69, 73, 75, 79, 81
Psaltriparus minimus, 99
public health, viii, 2, 28
public health policy, viii, 2
purification, 69, 70, 89, 90

R

rainfall, viii, 2, 4, 6, 8, 24, 26, 28, 42, 95
receptor, viii, 68, 69, 76, 80
recombinant protein, viii, 67, 68, 69, 76, 80, 87, 89, 90
recombinant proteins, viii, 67, 68, 69, 80
recovery, ix, 10, 12, 28, 45, 46, 47, 48, 49, 50, 51, 94, 100, 101, 102, 103, 107
reproduction, 11, 27, 41, 53
response, 57, 73, 75, 76, 77, 78, 80, 103
risk, viii, 2, 28, 56, 80, 99, 103, 104
roadside surveys, 100

S

Sacramento, 93, 95, 97, 98, 99, 100, 104, 108
safety, 73, 76
San Francisco Bay estuary, 95
San Joaquin valley, 95

science, 34, 61
scope, 6, 11, 42, 53
sensitivity, ix, 53, 71, 94
serum, 70, 71, 73, 77, 80
showing, 7, 97, 99, 101, 102
signs, ix, 49, 93, 101, 102
simulation, 5, 11, 12, 13, 14, 15, 16, 17, 18, 19, 20, 21, 24, 28, 30, 53, 56, 60
Sitta carolinensis, 99
species, vii, ix, 2, 3, 4, 5, 6, 8, 10, 11, 12, 14, 26, 28, 30, 31, 40, 44, 45, 46, 47, 48, 49, 50, 51, 64, 93, 94, 95, 99, 101, 102, 103, 104, 107
structural protein, viii, 67
structure, 4, 27, 31, 40
Sun, 37, 85
surveillance, 11, 42, 71, 105
survival, vii, ix, 75, 94
susceptibility, 44, 105
symptoms, 3, 49

T

tar, viii, 2, 6, 15, 36, 39, 41, 44, 46, 56, 62, 63, 64, 65, 66
temperature, viii, 2, 4, 6, 8, 11, 19, 24, 26, 27, 28, 41, 42, 56, 70
test data, 15, 17, 52
training, 15, 16, 17, 52
traits, 3, 31, 41
transgenic plant, viii, 67, 68, 69, 78, 80
transmission, 2, 3, 4, 8, 10, 12, 27, 30, 37, 40, 41, 44, 45, 106

V

vaccine, viii, 67, 68, 69, 72, 73, 74, 75, 76, 77, 78, 79, 80, 81, 82, 83, 84, 85, 86, 87, 88, 89, 90
validation, 15, 27, 28, 52
variables, 10, 11, 56
variations, 11, 12, 15, 16, 42, 55, 57
vector, 3, 12, 13, 40, 44, 75
virus infection, 69, 77, 78, 80, 105, 106, 107
virus-resistant, 103

W

water, 26, 40, 56, 59
West Nile virus, v, vii, viii, ix, 1, 2, 31, 32, 33, 34, 35, 36, 37, 38, 39, 43, 60, 61, 62, 63, 64, 65, 66, 67, 68, 69, 74, 77, 78, 80, 81, 82, 83, 84, 85, 86, 87, 88, 89, 90, 91, 93, 94, 102, 104, 105, 106, 107, 108
wetlands, 41, 56
white-breasted nuthatch, 99
worldwide, 71, 80

Y

yellow-billed magpie, v, vii, ix, 93, 94, 95, 98, 99, 100, 101, 102, 103, 104, 105, 106, 107, 108

Zika Virus Disease: Prevention and Cure

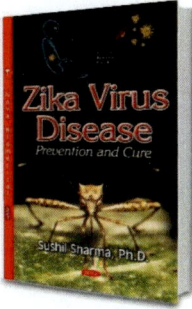

Author: Sushil K. Sharma, Ph.D.

Series: Virology Research Progress

Book Description: The author was motivated to write this important book because currently there is no systematically-written document on the ZIKV disease, which could serve at this crucial moment as a textbook for medical students, physicians, nurses, and other healthcare providers as well as a reference book for basic researchers, professors, and the general public.

Hardcover ISBN: 978-1-53610-769-2
Retail Price: $230

Dengue Virus: Detection, Diagnosis and Control

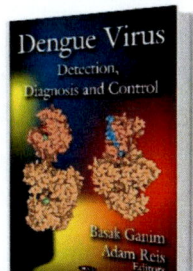

Editors: Basak Ganim and Adam Reis

Series: Virology Research Progress

Book Description: This book aims to review the possible molecular mechanisms that attribute to the variation of Dengue virus (DENV) disease.

Hardcover ISBN: 978-1-60876-398-6
Retail Price: $280

Viral Infections: Causes, Treatment Options and Potential Complications

Editor: Deborah Shinn

Series: Virology Research Progress

Book Description: This book discusses several topics that include viral infections in obstetrics and gynecology; the management of HIV infection by Chinese medicine; antiviral activity of lactoferrin; and antiviral effects of phytochemicals of the Mediterranean medicinal plants.

Hardcover ISBN: 978-1-63117-221-2
Retail Price: $179